Managing Women's Hyperandrogenism

Mariagrazia Stracquadanio

Managing Women's Hyperandrogenism

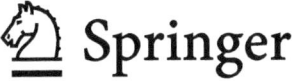 Springer

Mariagrazia Stracquadanio
Complex Operative Unit Obstetrics and Gynecology
Maria Paternò Arezzo Hospital
Contrada Rito
Ragusa
Italy

ISBN 978-3-030-29222-5   ISBN 978-3-030-29223-2   (eBook)
https://doi.org/10.1007/978-3-030-29223-2

This Springer imprint is published by the registered company Springer Nature Switzerland AG
The registered company address is: Gewerbestrasse 11, 6330 Cham, Switzerland

I dedicate this book to my son Gabriele and my husband Giancarlo.

Acknowledgments

A special thanks goes to my advisor Prof. Lilliana Ciotta (University of Catania), who has been a constant guide in the complex world of gynecological endocrinology.

Contents

Chapter 1
Definition
and Epidemiology

Androgen excess is the most common endocrine disorder in women of reproductive age. Some authors consider "hirsutism" as the result of an atypical relationship between levels of circulating androgens and the sensitivity of androgen receptors in hair follicles to circulating androgens [1].

Androgens are mainly produced by adrenal glands and ovaries. However, peripheral tissues such as fat and skin also play important roles in converting weak androgens to more potent ones. Androgen excess can affect different tissues and organs, causing variable clinical features such as acne, hirsutism, virilization, and reproductive dysfunction [2].

Androgen synthesis is regulated via the alteration of gene transcription by LH and ACTH of the anterior pituitary gland. The increase in androgen production in women, observed after the mid-cycle LH surge, is regulated by cholesterol access to the mitochondria via activation of steroidogenic acute regulatory protein (StAR) [3, 4].

In the target tissues, androgens enter the cell cytoplasm through simple diffusion across the cell membrane. Once inside the cell, androgens bind and activate the androgen receptors. The androgen–receptor complex attaches to a specific DNA site and stimulates the production of messenger RNA, which, in turn, stimulates the production of the enzymes and proteins necessary to affect androgen action.

© Springer Nature Switzerland AG 2020
M. Stracquadanio, *Managing Women's Hyperandrogenism*,
https://doi.org/10.1007/978-3-030-29223-2_1

Ovaries produce 25% of circulating testosterone and also secrete 50% of the androstenedione and 20% of DHEA. Testosterone is used as a marker of ovarian androgen secretion; however, the adrenals also contribute to circulating testosterone via peripheral conversion of androstenedione to testosterone.

On the other hand, the adrenal glands produce all of the DHEAS and 80% of the DHEA. The adrenals also secrete 50% of androstenedione and 25% of circulating testosterone. DHEAS and 11-androstenedione are not secreted by the ovaries and, therefore, are used as markers of adrenal androgen secretion. Moreover, both prolactin and estrogen can affect adrenal androgen production.

Skin, fat, liver, and urogenital systems are important peripheral sites of androgen production. Androstenedione and DHEA are converted to testosterone in the skin.

Only testosterone and DHT (dihydrotestosterone) are able to activate androgen receptors.

In women, the major circulating androgens are (in order of descending serum concentration) DHEAS, DHEA, androstenedione, testosterone (T), and DHT. However, only T and DHT have strong affinity and potency for the androgen receptor [1, 5].

In reproductive-aged women, 25% of the circulating testosterone derives from the adrenals and 25% is produced by the ovaries. The rest of the testosterone is produced by the peripheral conversion of androstenedione in adipose tissue. In healthy women, 80% of testosterone is bound to sex hormone-binding globulin (SHBG), 19% is bound to albumin, and 1% freely circulates in the bloodstream. The androgenicity depends mainly on the unbound fraction due to the high affinity of SHBG to the bound androgens. The levels of SHBG depend on several conditions and medications. For example, SHBG levels are increased by estrogens, thyroid hormones, and pregnancy, while they are decreased by androgens, synthetic progestins, glucocorticoids, insulin, and obesity. DHEAS, DHEA, and androstenedione are almost entirely bound to albumin. Unlike SHBG, albumin has a low affinity for sex hormones, so the albumin-bound androgens are readily available to tissues.

The clearance of androgens is accomplished by hepatic extraction and peripheral metabolism; most of the circulating T is metabolized via hepatic conjugation with glucuronic or sulfuric acids or voided as 17-ketosteroids in urine [5,6].The metabolism and clearance of circulating androgens may be altered by age, presence of obesity, medical conditions, and medications.

Androgens induce virilization and are responsible for forming the male external genitalia in the fetus. Moreover, they induce the growth of sexual hair, temporal balding, acne, clitoral growth, sebum production, and a deepening of the voice.

Androgens have direct effects on different body systems and also act as precursor hormones for ovarian and extragonadal estrogen synthesis. Androgen receptors are present in a variety of tissues like skeletal muscles, skin, gastrointestinal tract, genitourinary tract, bone, brain, cardiovascular system, placenta, and adipose tissues. Androgen actions are not completely understood in all of these tissues [7].

Androgen receptors are distributed throughout the brain in close proximity to estrogen receptors. The highest concentrations are present in the preoptic area of the hypothalamus. Some areas contain 5α-reductase and aromatase and are able to convert testosterone to DHT or estradiol [8]. Androgen can have activational behavior on women and may have some negative effects on the cognitive functions of older women [9].

Growing evidence supports the role of androgens in physiologic levels and sexual desire. Decreased sexual function has been reported in hyperandrogenic women receiving antiandrogens; on the other hand, administration of testosterone in women with hypoactive sexual desire disorder results in improvements in libido and sexual function [10, 11].

Androgens have important roles in bone mineralization either directly or through aromatization to estrogen. Lower androgen concentrations have been associated with bone loss in various age groups [12].

Androgen receptors are present in mammary epithelial cells in addition to estrogen and progesterone receptors. The proposed mechanisms include either direct stimulation of the androgen receptors or conversion to estradiol by the aromatase enzyme present in breast tissue. Androgens, particularly DHEA and testosterone, have been reported to protect against mammary epithelial proliferation in female monkeys. The reverse effect was reported when the anti-androgen flutamide was given to those animals [13].

Few data are available regarding the effects of androgens on human breasts. Hyperandrogenemia in women with polycystic ovary syndrome (PCOS) does not appear to have significant risk of breast cancer [14]. In a prospective randomized controlled study in postmenopausal women evaluating breast cell proliferation and testosterone, the authors found no significant difference when testosterone was added to estrogen and progesterone, while they found a fivefold increase in breast cell proliferation in women taking the placebo [15].

Unopposed estrogen stimulation of the endometrium increases the risk of endometrial hyperplasia and eventually cancer. The proposed mechanism of androgen aromatization to estradiol may not be applicable because the aromatase expression has not been detected in normal endometrium and stromal cells [16]. In vitro studies have shown that androgens have an inhibitory effect on endometrial proliferation [17].

There is a great concern about the relation between sex hormones and cardiovascular events. Women with PCOS have hyperandrogenemia and are at higher risk of cardiovascular events [18–20]. However, the insulin resistance associated with PCOS is likely more relevant to the pathogenesis of cardiovascular disease. Moreover, the exogenous administration of testosterone for female-to-male transsexual has not been associated with the increased risk of cardiovascular disease [21].

In the target tissues, androgens enter the cell cytoplasm by simple diffusion across the cell membrane. Once inside the cell, the androgens bind and activate the androgen receptors.

The androgen–receptor complex attaches to a specific DNA site and stimulates the production of messenger RNA, which, in turn, stimulates the production of the enzymes and proteins necessary to affect androgen action.

The prevalence of androgen excess among US population is 8%.

The international incidence rate is dependent on the particular culture, but, essentially, it is similar to that of the United States.

A recent Italian study, conducted in a large population of high-school students in Northern Italy, showed an incidence of 24% of girls with isolated clinical hyperandrogenism and 8% of female students affected by PCOS [22].

In premenopausal African-American women, relative androgen excess is associated with insulin resistance and increased risk for development of type 2 diabetes [23].

Impaired glucose tolerance and type 2 diabetes affect about 40% of women with PCOS. The presence of PCOS is an independent cardiovascular risk factor. Women who have anovulatory PCOS have greater cardiovascular risk compared with women who have ovulatory PCOS and idiopathic hyperandrogenism.

Androgen-secreting tumors are rare and about 30% of them are malignant.

Androgen excess occurs equally in all races. Congenital adrenal hyperplasia prevalence due to 21-hydroxylase deficiency is greater among those of Ashkenazi Jewish descent.

The most common causes of hyperandrogenism begin in early adolescence or in childbearing age. Androgen-producing tumors may rarely affect postmenopausal women.

Some authors have reported that the development of the disorder is under genetic control, although the mode of transmission is unclear. Data from an old study [24] suggest that PCOS, for example, is a familial disorder, with a single autosomal dominant gene effect, that presents with a variable phenotype; inheritance appears to be equally probable from the maternal as from the paternal side of the family.

References

1. Blume-Peytavi HS. Medical treatment of hirsutism. Dermatol Ther. 2008;21:329–39.
2. Azziz R, Nestler JE, Dewailly D. Androgen excess disorders in women: polycystic ovary syndrome and other disorders, vol. XVIII. Totowa, NJ: Humana Press; 2006, 46pp.
3. Lizneva D, Gavrilova-Jordan L, Walker W, et al. Androgen excess: investigation and management. Best Pract Res Clin Obstet Gynec. 2016;37:98–118.
4. Stocco DM, Clark BJ. Regulation of the acute production of steroids in steroidogenic cells. Endocr Rev. 1996;17(3):221–44.
5. Longcope C. Adrenal and gonadal androgen secretion in normal females. Clin Endocrinol Metab. 1986;15(2):213–28.
6. Juricskay S, Telegdy E. Urinary steroids in women with androgenic alopecia. Clin Biochem. 2000;33(2):97–101.
7. Davison SL, Bell R. Androgen physiology. Semin Reprod Med. 2006;24(2):71–7.
8. Schiffer L, Kempegowda P, Arlt W, O'Reilly MW. Mechanisms in endocrinology: the sexually dimorphic role of androgens in human metabolic disease. Eur J Endocrinol. 2017;177(3):R125–43.
9. Baulieu EE. Neurosteroids: a novel function of the brain. Psychoneuroendocrinology. 1998;23(8):963–87.
10. Hogervorst E, Matthews FE, Brayne C. Are optimal levels of testosterone associated with better cognitive function in healthy older women and men? Biochim Biophys Acta. 2010;1800(10):1145–52.
11. Appelt H, Strauss B. Effects of antiandrogen treatment on the sexuality of women with hyperandrogenism. Psychother Psychosom. 1984;42(1–4):177–81.
12. Buster JE, Kingsberg SA, Aguirre O, Brown C, Breaux JG, Buch A, et al. Testosterone patch for low sexual desire in surgically menopausal women: a randomized trial. Obstet Gynecol. 2005;105(5 Pt 1):944–52.
13. Slemenda C, Longcope C, Peacock M, Hui S, Johnston CC. Sex steroids, bone mass, and bone loss. A prospective study of pre-, peri-, and postmenopausal women. J Clin Invest. 1996;97(1):14–21.
14. Dimitrakakis C, Zhou J, Wang J, Belanger A, LaBrie F, Cheng C, et al. A physiologic role for testosterone in limiting estrogenic stimulation of the breast. Menopause. 2003;10(4):292–8.
15. Anderson KE, Sellers TA, Chen PL, Rich SS, Hong CP, Folsom AR. Association of Stein-Leventhal syndrome with the inci-

dence of postmenopausal breast carcinoma in a large prospective study of women in Iowa. Cancer. 1997;79(3):494–9.

16. Hofling M, Hirschberg AL, Skoog L, Tani E, Hagerstrom T, von Schoultz B. Testosterone inhibits estrogen/progestogen-induced breast cell proliferation in postmenopausal women. Menopause. 2007;14(2):183–90.

17. Bulun SE, Mahendroo MS, Simpson ER. Polymerase chain reaction amplification fails to detect aromatase cytochrome P450 transcripts in normal human endometrium or decidua. J Clin Endocrinol Metab. 1993;76(6):1458–63.

18. Tuckerman EM, Okon MA, Li T, Laird SM. Do androgens have a direct effect on endometrial function? An in vitro study. Fertil Steril. 2000;74(4):771–9.

19. Talbott E, Guzick D, Clerici A, Berga S, Detre K, Weimer K, et al. Coronary heart disease risk factors in women with polycystic ovary syndrome. Arterioscler Thromb Vasc Biol. 1995;15(7):821–6.

20. Ehrmann DA, Schneider DJ, Sobel BE, Cavaghan MK, Imperial J, Rosenfield RL, et al. Troglitazone improves defects in insulin action, insulin secretion, ovarian steroidogenesis, and fibrinolysis in women with polycystic ovary syndrome. J Clin Endocrinol Metab. 1997;82(7):2108–16.

21. Holte J, Gennarelli G, Wide L, Lithell H, Berne C. High prevalence of polycystic ovaries and associated clinical, endocrine, and metabolic features in women with previous gestational diabetes mellitus. J Clin Endocrinol Metab. 1998;83(4):1143–50.

22. Gambineri A, Prontera O, Fanelli F, et al. Epidemiological survey on the prevalence of hyperandrogenic states in adolescent and young women. Endocr Abstr. 2012;29:OC16.4.

23. Boyd-Woschinko G, Kushner H, Falkner B. Androgen excess is associated with insulin resistance and the development of diabetes in African American women. J Cardiometab Syndr. 2007;2(4):254–9.

24. Kashar-Miller M, Azziz R. Heritability and the risk of developing androgen excess. J Steroid Biochem Mol Biol. 1999;69:261–8.

Chapter 2
Causes of Hyperandrogenism

The differential diagnosis of the hyperandrogenic patient includes idiopathic hirsutism, polycystic ovary syndrome (PCOS), the hyperandrogenic insulin-resistant acanthosis nigricans (HAIRAN) syndrome, 21-hydroxylase-deficient non-classic congenital adrenal hyperplasia or classic congenital adrenal hyperplasia, and androgen-secreting neoplasm. Rare causes include side effects from medication, hypothyroidism, hyperprolactinemia, and Cushing's disease [1, 2].

2.1   Ovarian Diseases: PCOS

Polycystic ovary syndrome (PCOS) is a heterogeneous endocrine and metabolic disorder, characterized by chronic anovulation/ oligomenorrhea, hyperandrogenism, and insulin resistance [3]. In PCOS, in fact, we can distinguish two sides of the same coin: endocrine and metabolic aspects [4].

PCOS is a multifactorial polygenic disease (interaction between several genetic and environmental factors), with a heritability of ~70%. It is intrinsically difficult to study by a genetic point of view, and most of the current literature

© Springer Nature Switzerland AG 2020
M. Stracquadanio, *Managing Women's Hyperandrogenism*,
https://doi.org/10.1007/978-3-030-29223-2_2

(>70 studies based on the candidate gene approach) is inconclusive, with many studies resulting inconsistent, controversial, and without a clear consensus [5].

Even if several studies conducted in families of women with PCOS have demonstrated the genetic basis of the syndrome, nowadays a genetic pattern certainly involved in PCOS predisposition has not been identified.

Most studies have included different kinds of genes: those related to androgen biosynthesis and action and their regulation, genes involved in insulin resistance and associated disorders, and also genes involved in chronic inflammation and atherosclerosis.

More than 80% of women showing symptoms of androgen excess have PCOS [6]. The main symptoms of hyperandrogenism are acne/seborrhea, hirsutism, and defluvium/alopecia.

Hyperandrogenemia is the biochemical features of PCOS. Elevated circulating androgen levels are observed in 80–90% of women with oligomenorrhea [7].

In particular, it is reported a decreased SHBG (sex hormone binding globulin) production with a consequent increase in free testosterone levels. Furthermore, some authors suggest that, vice versa, SHBG levels are decreased in PCOS due to the effects of testosterone and insulin to decrease hepatic production of SHBG [8, 9].

Ovaries are the main sources of increased androgens in PCOS, but even adrenal androgen excess is a common feature of the syndrome (approximately 20% of PCOS women): it was demonstrated an increased secretion of adrenocortical precursor steroids basally and in response to ACTH, such as pregnenolone, 17-hydroxyprogesterone (17-OH-P), dehydroepiandrosterone (DHEA), and androstenedione (A) [10, 11].

It has been suggested that androgens enhance apoptosis in the granulosa cells of preantral and early antral follicles [12]. Moreover, a study found that the exposure to excessive androstenedione stimulates a premature luteinization of granulosa cells, most likely due to the loss of communication between the oocyte and the granulosa cell [13].

Due to the pulsatility of LH, only one blood parameter is not enough for the PCOS diagnosis, and there is no unanimous consensus on which androgen blood levels should be considered for a precise diagnosis (total or free testosterone, testosterone/SHBG ratio, or androstenedione). Usually, elevated levels of only DHEA or 17-OHP may exclude the diagnosis of PCOS [14].

Hyperinsulinemia also contributes to the high androgen levels: indeed, insulin resistance, and consequent compensatory hyperinsulinemia, appears to be the central pathophysiologic mechanism that links PCOS to its metabolic disorders; in fact, few studies reported that PCOS women are more insulin resistant than controls who are matched for age and BMI [15]. High level of insulin accelerates the development of granulosa cells LH responsiveness by amplifying the induction of LH receptors, and, thus, it induces a block of follicular growth with multiple small follicles formation.

Some authors have shown that fasting hyperinsulinemia in PCOS women is the result of a combination of increased basal insulin secretion and decreased hepatic insulin clearance [16, 17].

Lots of evidence demonstrates a direct insulin action on ovarian steroidogenesis and the importance of the insulin-signaling pathway in the control of ovulation.

The central paradox in the pathophysiologic association between hyperinsulinemia and hyperandrogenemia in PCOS is that the ovary remains sensitive to insulin activity and consequent androgen production, despite a systemic insulin resistance: it is the so-called *selective insulin resistance* theory [18].

On the other hand, androgens can produce insulin resistance by direct effects on skeletal muscle and adipose tissue insulin action, by altering adipokine secretion, and by increasing visceral adiposity, even if these effects on insulin actions are modest [19].

The correlation between PCOS, insulin, hyperandrogenism, and ovarian dysfunction is well exemplified in Fig. 2.1.

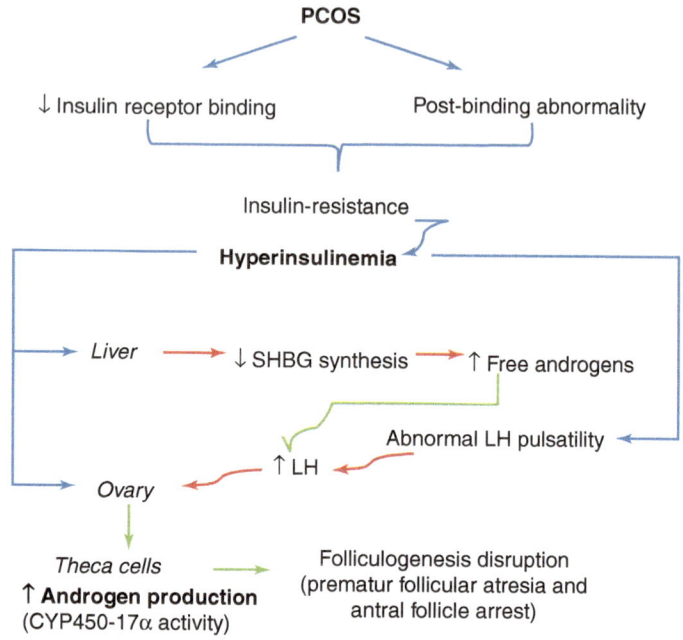

Figure 2.1 Correlation between PCOS, hyperinsulinemia, hyperandrogenism, and ovarian dysfunction [4]

2.2 Non-classic Adrenal Hyperplasia (NCAH)

NCAH is encountered with relatively high frequency (1–6%) among adolescent and adult patients with hyperandrogenism. This incidence may vary from one geographic area to another due to different ethnic and racial clusters [20].

The 21-hydroxylase deficiency is responsible for an oversecretion of 17-OHP and other steroids that are upstream this enzymatic step. Gene mutations of cytochrome P450 C21, resulting in NCAH, reduce the activity of 21-hydroxylase to 20–50%. This is not sufficient to impair the physiologically needed cortisol production, thus compensating for the lower enzyme efficiency. The alteration in the enzyme kinetic explains the excessive accumulation of 21-OH precursors, mainly progesterone and 17 OHP, in the presence of a normal stimulation by ACTH. This excess is partly converted to androgens, resulting in adrenal hyperandrogenism.

Cytochrome P450 C21 gene is localized on chromosome 6. In NCAH, the most frequent mutation is V281L. Patients are homozygote or compound heterozygote with another mutation sometimes severe on the other allele. Considering the high frequency of heterozygote in the general population, it is essential to genotype the partner of the patient to offer eventual genetic counselling [20, 21].

In summary, hyperandrogenism in NCAH results from:

– Adrenal hyperactivity depending on altered enzyme kinetics without increased ACTH circulating levels
– Increased peripheral conversion to androgens of circulating excessive levels of steroid metabolites
– Increased ovarian androgen secretion determined by the appearance of a secondary PCOS-like phenotype in NCAH patients [22]

Before the age of 7–8 years, NCAH may mimic an idiopathic premature pubarche; several studies have shown that adolescent or adult women with NCAH are more virilized than other women with ovarian causes of hyperandrogenism [23]: they generally present with hirsutism, acne, and/or androgenic alopecia; clitoromegaly has been reported in 6–20% of adult women with NCAH. Moreover, 30–50% of patients with NCAH show ovulatory and menstrual dysfunction [24]. Even though adrenal hyperplasia and adenomas have been reported in patients with NCAH, the real prevalence of this pathology remains unknown [22].

2.3 Adrenal and Ovarian Tumors

These causes of hyperandrogenism are rare. The clinical presentation is often suggestive: symptoms of deep virilization such as increased libido, deepened voice, and clitoromegaly. The laboratory investigations will show high androgen levels and rapidly confirm the clinical suspicion, while imaging techniques will localize the tumor [20].

2.4   Cushing Syndrome (CS)

Cushing syndrome is caused by prolonged exposure to high circulating levels of cortisol. There are two main etiologies of Cushing syndrome: endogenous hypercortisolism and exogenous hypercortisolism. Exogenous hypercortisolism, the most common cause of Cushing syndrome, is mostly iatrogenic and results from the prolonged use of glucocorticoids. Endogenous Cushing syndrome results from excessive production of cortisol by adrenal glands and can be ACTH-dependent and ACTH-independent. ACTH-secreting pituitary adenomas (Cushing disease) and ectopic ACTH secretion by neoplasms are responsible for ACTH-dependent Cushing. Adrenal hyperplasia, adenoma, and carcinoma are major causes of ACTH-independent Cushing syndrome [25–27].

Cortisol is a steroid hormone produced by the zona fasciculata of the adrenal cortex. After production the cortisol is carried to different parts of the body by cortisol binding protein, almost 90% of cortisol binds to these (CBG) proteins and has a bioavailability of 60–100%. Synthetic corticosteroids have varying bioavailability and potency but all affect similar pathways. It is a catabolic hormone which is released under stressful conditions. The excess of cortisol results in an increased rate of gluconeogenesis and glycogenolysis and increases insulin resistance. Cortisol is a steroid hormone, and it directly affects the transcription and translation of enzyme proteins involved in the metabolism of fats, glycogen, protein synthesis, and Kreb's cycle. It promotes the production of free glucose in the body, elevating glucose levels, while simultaneously increasing insulin resistance [28].

Physical examination of the patient will reveal increased fat deposits in the upper half of the body leading to "Buffalo torso," characteristic moon facies (earlobes are not visible when viewed from the front), thin arms and legs, acne, hirsutism, proximal muscle weakness of shoulder and hip girdle muscles, paper-thin skin, abdominal pain due to gut perforation in rare cases, and wide vertical purplish abdominal striae.

The evaluation of suspected Cushing's syndrome can include the demonstration of endogenous hypercortisolism with the late-night salivary cortisol or a 24-h urine-free cortisol [29].

Routine screening for CS in patients with a referral diagnosis of hirsutism is not required. Diagnostic tests for Cushing syndrome in hirsute patients cannot be recommended if the patient does not have clinical stigmata of hypercortisolism [30].

2.5   Hyperprolactinemia

Prolactin excess stimulates the secretion of adrenal androgens, mainly DHEAS. Therefore, a mild hyperandrogenism frequently accompanies the clinical expression of a prolactinoma, but it is rarely the main complaint [20].

2.6   Drugs

Drugs are the most commonly responsible for the development of virilizing effects that include anabolic steroids, nortestosterone-derived progestins, and antiepileptic drugs [20]. Hirsutism and androgenic alopecia must be differentiated from drug-induced hypertrichosis or hair loss, which are independent from hormone stimulation [31].

2.7   Idiopathic Hirsutism (IH)

IH is defined as hirsutism associated with normal ovulatory function and normal serum androgen levels [32]. Its pathogenesis is not clear: increased peripheral 5a-reductase activity and androgen receptor gene polymorphism could lead to this disease [33–35]. Indeed, estradiol/testosterone ratio, which is a function of aromatase activity, was also found to be lower in patients with IH [36]. On the other hand, human skin presents all the enzymes necessary for androgen synthesis and catabolism indicating that it is an independent peripheral endocrine organ [37]. The cutaneous expressions of steroidogenic acute regulatory protein, cytochrome P450 cholesterol sidechain cleavage (P450scc), and cytochrome P450 17-alpha hydroxylase (P450c17) have been demonstrated previously which suggest that the cutaneously derived cholesterol could be further used as a substrate for de novo steroid hormone synthesis in human epidermis and the sebaceous gland [38].

References

1. Azziz R, Sanchex LA, Knochenhauer ES, et al. Androgen excess in women: experience with over 1000 consecutive patients. J Clin Endocrinol Metab. 2004;89(2):453–62.
2. Legro RS, Arslanian SA, Ehrmann DA, et al. Diagnosis and treatment of polycystic ovary syndrome: and Endocrine Society Clinical Practice guideline. J Clin Endocrinol Metab. 2013;98(12):4565–92.
3. Rotterdam ESHRE/ASRM-Sponsored PCOS Consensus Workshop Group. Revised. Consensus on diagnostic criteria and long- term health risks related to polycystic ovary syndrome. Fertil Steril. 2003;81:19–25.
4. Stracquadanio M, Ciotta L. Metabolic aspects of PCOS. 2015. ISBN 978-3-319-16759-6.
5. Barber TM, Franks S. Genetics of polycystic ovary syndrome. Front Horm Res. 2013;40:28–39.
6. Diaz A, Laufer MR, Breech LL. Menstruation in girls and adolescents: using the menstrual cycle as a vital sign. Pediatrics. 2006;118(5):2245–50.
7. Azziz R, Task Force on the Phenotype of the Polycystic Ovary Syndrome of the Androgen Excess PCOS Society et al. The androgen excess and PCOS society criteria for the polycystic ovary syndrome: the complete task force report. Fertil Steril. 2009;91:456–88.
8. Molli GW Jr, Rosenfield RL. Testosterone binding and free plasma androgen concentrations under physiological conditions: characterization by flow dialysis technique. J Clin Endocrinol Metab. 1979;49:730–6.

9. Nestler JE, Powers LP, Matt DW, et al. A direct effect of hyper-insulinemia on serum sex hormone-binding globulin levels in obese women with the polycystic ovary syndrome. J Clin Endocrinol Metab. 1991;72:83–9.

10. Yildiz BO, Azziz R. The adrenal and polycystic ovary syndrome. Rev Endocr Metab Disord. 2007;8:331–42.

11. Lachelin GC, Barnett M, Hopper BR, et al. Adrenal function in normal women and women with the polycystic ovary syndrome. J Clin Endocrinol Metab. 1979;49:892–8.

12. Billing H, Furuta I, Hsueh AJW. Estrogens inhibit and andro-gen enhance ovarian granulosa cell apoptosis. Endocrinology. 1993;133:2204–12.

13. Okutsu Y, et al. Exogenous androstenedione induces formation of follicular cysts and premature luteinization of granulosa cells in the ovary. Fertil Steril. 2010;93:927–35.

14. Ciotta L, Stracquadanio M, et al. Effects of Myo-inositol supple-mentation on oocyte's quality in PCOS patients: a double blind trial. Eur Rev Med Pharmacol Sci. 2011;15:509–14.

15. Hoffman LK, Ehrmann DA. Cardiometabolic features of poly-cystic ovary syndrome. Nat Clin Pract Endocrinol Metab. 2008;4(4):215–22.

16. O'Meara NM, Blackman JD, Ehrmann DA, et al. Defects in β-cell function in functional ovarian hyperandrogenism. J Clin Endocrinol Metab. 1993;76:1241–7.

17. Peiris AN, Mueller RA, Struve MF, et al. Relationship of andro-genic activity to splanchnic insulin metabolism and peripheral glucose utilization in premenopausal women. J Clin Endocrinol Metab. 1987;64:162–9.

18. Book C, Dunaif A. Selective insulin resistance in the polycystic ovary syndrome. J Clin Endocrinol Metab. 1999;84(9):3110–6.

19. Diamanti-Kandarakis E, Dunaif A. Insulin resistance and the polycystic ovary syndrome revisited: an update on mechanisms and implications. Endocr Rev. 2012;33(6):981–1030.

20. Catteau-Jonard S, Cortet Rudelli C, et al. Hyperandrogenism in adolescent girls. Endocr Dev. 2012;22:181–93.

21. Bidet M, Bellanne-Chantelot C, Galand-Portier MB, et al. Clinical and molecular characterization of a cohort of 161 unre-lated women with non-classical congenital adrenal hyperplasia due to 21-hydroxylase deficiency and 330 family members. J Clin Endocrinol Metab. 2009;94:1570–8.

22. Carmina E, Dewailly D, Escobar-Morreale H, et al. Non-classic congenital adrenal hyperplasia due to 21-hydroxylase deficiency

revisited: an update with a special focus on adolescent and adult women. Hum Reprod Update. 2017;23(5):580–99.

23. Moran C, Azziz R, Carmina E, et al. 21-Hydroxylase-deficient nonclassic adrenal hyperplasia is a progressive disorder: a multicenter study. Am J Obstet Gynecol. 2000;183:1468–74.

24. Akinci A, Yordam N, Ersoy F, et al. The incidence of non-classical 21-hydroxylase deficiency in hirsute adolescent girls. Gynecol Endocrinol. 1992;6:99–106.

25. Osswald A, Deutschbein T, Berr CM, et al. Surviving ectopic Cushing's syndrome: quality of life, cardiovascular and metabolic outcomes in comparison to Cushing's disease during long-term follow-up. Eur J Endocrinol. 2018;179(2):109–16.

26. Zhao Y, Guo H, Zhao Y, Shi B. Secreting ectopic adrenal adenoma: a rare condition to be aware of. Ann Endocrinol. 2018;79(2):75–81.

27. O'Brien KF, DeKlotz CMC, Silverman RA. Exogenous Cushing syndrome from an unexpected source of systemic steroids. Pediatr Dermatol. 2018;35(3):e196–7.

28. Moreira AC, Antonini SR, de Castro M. Mechanisms in endocrinology: a sense of time of the glucocorticoid circadian clock: from the ontogeny to the diagnosis of Cushing's syndrome. Eur J Endocrinol. 2018;179(1):R1–R18.

29. Nieman LK, Biller BM, Findling JW, et al. The diagnosis of Cushing's syndrome: an Endocrine Society Clinical Practice Guideline. J Clin Endocrinol Metab. 2008;93(5):1526–40.

30. Karaca Z, Acmaz B, Acmaz G, et al. Routine screening for Cushing's syndrome is not required in patients presenting with hirsutism. Eur J Endocrinol. 2013;168:379–84.

31. Cortet-Rudelli C, Desailloud R, Dewailly D. Drug-induced androgen excess. In: Azziz R, Nestler JE, Dewailly D, editors. Androgen excess disorders in women. Philadelphia: Raven Press-Lippincott; 1997. p. 613–22.

32. Azziz R, Carmina E, Sawaya ME. Idiopathic hirsutism. Endocr Rev. 2000;21:347–62.

33. Serafini P, Lobo RA. Increased 5-α-reductase activity in idiopathic hirsutism. Fertil Steril. 1985;43:74–8.

34. Sawaya ME, Shalita AR. Androgen receptor polymorphism (CAG repeat lengths) in androgenetic alopecia, hirsutism and acne. J Cutan Med Surg. 1998;3:9–15.

35. Legro RS, Shahbahrami B, Lobo RA, et al. Size polymorphisms of the androgen receptor among female Hispanics and

correlations with androgenic characteristics. Obstet Gynecol. 1994;83:701–6.

36. Unluhizarci K, Karababa Y, et al. The investigation of insulin resistance in patients with idiopathic hirsutism. J Clin Endocrinol Metab. 2004;89:2741–4.

37. Taheri S, Zararsiz G, Karaburgu S, et al. Is idiopathic hirsutism (IH) really idiopathic? mRNA expressions of skin steroidogenic enzymes in women with IH. Eur J Endocrinol. 2015;173:447–54.

38. Chen W, Thiboutot D, Zouboulis CC. Cutaneous androgen metabolism: basic research and clinical perspectives. J Invest Dermatol. 2002;119:992–1007.

Chapter 3
Clinical Features and Assessment of Hyperandrogenism: Differential Diagnosis for Clinical Use

Women hyperandrogenism can be clinically manifested (hirsutism, acne, alopecia, etc.) or biochemically evident through the measurements of blood androgens.

3.1 Biochemical Hyperandrogenism

Androgens circulate in the bloodstream in small amounts, and they are small steroidal molecules; thus it is important that the assays used for their detection be of the highest quality, such as high-quality radioimmunoassay (RIA) following sample extraction and chromatography.

Total testosterone levels are found to be elevated in 22–85% PCOS patients, while almost 70% of PCOS women have elevated serum concentration levels of free testosterone (FT), which is the single most sensitive test for hyperandrogenemia [1].

To diagnose biochemical hyperandrogenism is also useful the dosage of other androgens: for example, androstenedione is elevated in 18% of PCOS women. Moreover, the

© Springer Nature Switzerland AG 2020   21
M. Stracquadanio, *Managing Women's Hyperandrogenism*,
https://doi.org/10.1007/978-3-030-29223-2_3

measurement of DHEAS reflects adrenal androgen production: it is elevated in 25% of PCOS patients. It was found that the addition of DHEAS and androstenedione measures, when assessing patients with possible hyperandrogenism, each increases the percentage of patients considered "hyperandrogenic" [1].

3.2   Hirsutism

Hirsutism is defined as the presence of excessive terminal hairs in areas of the body that are androgen-dependent and usually hairless or with limited hair growth, such as face, chest, areolas, and abdomen [2].

Terminal hair is different from "vellus" hair, because the latter is the prolonged version of "lanugo" (the hair that covers fetuses and is shed gradually after birth) which covers all body surface except lips, palms, and soles; specifically, terminal hair is the pigmented, longer, coarser hair that covers the pubic and axillary areas, scalp, eyelashes, eyebrows, male body, and facial hair [3].

Hirsutism should be differentiated from hypertrichosis, which is the overgrowth of vellus in a nonsexual pattern distribution, usually related to persistence of the highly mitotic anagen phase of the hair cycle [4, 5].

Terminal hair growth requires androgen stimulation, especially testosterone and dihydrotestosterone (DHT) that can bind to the androgen receptor and promote hair follicle changes [3, 6].

Androgens, in fact, are the most significant hormones associated with hair growth modulation. They are necessary for terminal hair and sebaceous gland development and cause differentiation of pilosebaceous units into either a terminal hair follicle or a sebaceous gland. They are involved in keratinization, increased hair follicle size, hair fiber diameter, and the proportion of time that terminal hair spends in the anagen phase [7]. Androgens may act on hair follicles directly and/or independently on their serum levels, producing an intracrine or local effect [8, 9]. The control of hair growth and hair differentiation is established through local and circulating growth factors as transforming growth factor (EGF), stem cell factor (SCF), and vascular endothelial growth factor (VEGF) [10].

Thus, hyperandrogenemia is the cause of hirsutism, but the percentage of hair growth is not proportional to the degree of hyperandrogenism, supporting the important role for androgen receptor localization (keratinocytes, sebaceous glands, hair dermal papilla cells) and sensitivity in the development of hair patterns [11].

Hirsutism can be assessed through the Ferriman-Gallwey scale [12] that evaluates the presence of the terminal hair in the upper lip, chin, chest, upper and lower back, upper and lower abdomen, thighs, and arms.

A score of 0–4 is assigned to each area examined, based on the visual density of terminal hairs, such that a score of 0 represents the absence of terminal hairs, a score of 1 minimally evident terminal hair growth, and a score of 4 extensive terminal hair growth.

Integrated scores from all body areas beyond 15 points are related to a hirsutism diagnosis, although current recommendations suggest the use of 95th percentile of the score in specific populations, adapting to ethnic groups, hair pattern, and age-related features, in order to properly diagnose hirsutism [12].

For a correct evaluation, patients should be advised to avoid use of electrolysis or lasers for at least 3 months, depilation or waxing for 4 weeks, and not shaving at least 5 days prior to evaluation [13].

Some investigators [14–16] have classified patients with regular menstruation and hirsutism as having "idiopathic hirsutism (IH)", regardless of androgen levels.

On the other hand, hirsutism cannot be defined "idiopathic" if the excess hair growth arises consequent to an excess in circulating androgens [17].

Thus, it is more correct to define as having IH only when they are hirsute, normo-ovulatory, and euandrogenic [18].

This diagnosis is one of exclusion, and it is often observed in patients with a Mediterranean or Hispanic ethnic background. It is thought to result from increased skin 5α-reductase activity [19].

3.3   Acne

Sebaceous glands are also androgen-dependent structures: sebocytes are highly sensitive to androgen signaling, which is worsened in PCOS, leading to the development of acne and seborrhea [20].

Androgens stimulate sebocyte proliferation (particularly in the mid-back, chin, and forehead) and secretion of sebum, which is a mixture of lipids including glycerides, squalene, free fatty acids (FFA), and cholesterol [21].

Local bacteria complicate the process by secreting lipolytic enzymes: they break down those triglycerides produced in the sebocyte; these FFAs are released into sebaceous ducts by apocrine glands, and they are responsible for the typical unpleasant odor [22].

The two commonly used measures to assess the severity of acne are grading and lesion counting, but no grading system has been universally accepted [23].

In 1956, Pillsbury, Shelley, and Kligman published the earliest known grading system [24], which includes the following:

- Grade 1: comedones and occasional small cysts confined to the face.
- Grade 2: comedones with occasional pustules and small cysts confined to the face.
- Grade 3: many comedones and small and large inflammatory papules and pustules, more extensive but confined to the face.
- Grade 4: many comedones and deep lesions tending to coalescence and canalize and involving the face and the upper aspects of the trunk.

A more recent and complete system is the one created, in 1997, by Doshi et al. [25], called "Global Acne Grading System

(GAGS)." This system divides face, chest, and back into six areas (forehead, each cheek, nose, chin, chest, and back) and assigns a factor to each area on the basis of size.

Each type of lesion is given a value depending on severity:

- No lesions = 0.
- Comedones = 1.
- Papules = 2.
- Pustules = 3.
- Nodules = 4.

The score for each area (local score) is calculated using the formula:

$$\text{Local score} = \text{Factor} \times \text{Grade}\,(0-4).$$

The global score is the sum of local scores, and acne severity was graded using the global score. A score of 1–18 is considered mild; 19–30, moderate; 31–38, severe; and >39, very severe [26].

3.4   Alopecia: Female Pattern Hair Loss (FPHL)

An opposite clinical feature is androgenic alopecia that is a disorder characterized by miniaturized hair, due to an increased telogen/anagen ratio and associated to genetic susceptibility related to increased 5α-reductase activity in the hair follicle. This increased enzymatic activity promotes the local conversion of testosterone into DHT that has an increased androgen action [26].

FPHL is a thinning of hair primarily in the sagittal area of the scalp, caused by miniaturization of the hair follicles [1]. There are two common pattern types of FLP in women. Ludwig described diffuse hair thinning in the centroparietal region with a preserved frontal line. On the contrary, the "Christmas tree" pattern is associated with diffuse centroparietal

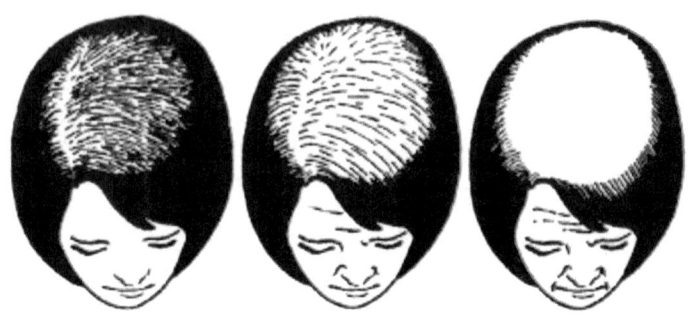

FIGURE 3.1 FPHL patterns [1, 27]

thinning of the hair with branching of the frontal hair line (Fig. 3.1) [27].

Moreover, evaluation should include an assessment of pattern distribution and the hair-pull test: it is an easy technique for assessing hair loss. Approximately 60 hairs are grasped between the thumb and the index and middle fingers; the hairs are then gently but firmly pulled. A negative test (6 or fewer hairs obtained) indicates normal shedding, whereas a positive test (more than 6 hairs obtained) indicates a process of active hair shedding. It is mandatory to advice the patient to not brush or wash her hair for 48 h before the exam. The use of photography of the affected area should be considered as a valid option for the follow-up [1].

FPHL is clinically diagnosed and it represents a diagnosis of exclusion. Exclusion of other causes of alopecia should be undertaken including tests to rule-out scalp fungal infections, autoimmune disorders, hematologic or nutritional defects, and systemic hyperandrogenism.

3.5   Hyperandrogenism in Adolescent Girls

Mild symptoms of hyperandrogenism, such as acne or hyperseborrhea, are very frequent in adolescent girls [28] and are often associated with irregular menstrual cycles. These symptoms are often transitory and only reflect the immaturity of the hypothalamic-pituitary-ovary axis during the first years following menarche [19].

At the beginning of puberty, LH pulsatility is only present during sleep; then, it extends to the daytime, with amplification of pulse amplitude and acceleration of frequency with a consequent increase of androgen plasma levels [19].

At the same time, there is a parallel change in the GH/IGF-1 axis, whose hyperactivity induces a selective insulin resistance, with a physiological hyperinsulinism and decreased SHBG levels.

Sometimes these signs can persist and hirsutism may appear, revealing an adrenal or ovarian disorder that is often caused by polycystic ovary syndrome (PCOS).

3.6 Diagnosis of Hyperandrogenism

The first visit must include a complete anamnesis and a careful physical examination. Clinical symptoms that must be searched for are the following:

- Rapidly growing hirsutism, with other signs of virilization such as clitoromegaly, temporal balding, voice deepening, and increasing muscle mass (they could be indicative of an adrenal or ovarian tumor).
- Symptoms of hypercorticism (in order to exclude Cushing syndrome).
- Galactorrhea, indicative of a prolactinoma.
- Hirsutism.
- Acne.
- Alopecia.
- Menstrual irregularities.
- Obesity or increased abdominal adiposity.
- Acanthosis nigricans.

The second step is to request a pelvic ultrasound (to know the presence of a polycystic ovarian morphology or ovarian tumor) and a laboratory screening.

Blood sampling must be performed early in the morning (to avoid false-negative results due to the circadian decrease in adrenal steroids that occurs later in the day) and during the early follicular phase of cycle to avoid false-positive results due to the steroid production from the corpus luteum. In amenorrheic or oligomeorrheic patients, blood sampling should be performed after a short sequence of progestin treatment. This laboratory screening must include the assay of total testosterone, DHEAS and 17-OHP, androstenedione, and prolactin.

The study group of Lille proposes an interesting flowchart (Fig. 3.2) for hyperandrogenism assessment [19].

If the 17 OHP value is >2 ng/mL (6 nmol/L), the nonclassic congenital adrenal 21-hydroxylase deficiency (NCAH) must be suspected, and ACTH test is required: it is an acute adrenal stimulation test that measures 17-OHP before and 60 min after the intravenous administration of an adrenocorticotropic hormone analog. If the stimulated 17-OHP exceeds 10 ng/mL (30 nmol/L), the diagnosis of NCAH is confirmed [29]. Thus, if this test is positive, it is recommended CYP2IA2 genotyping, with the aim of confirming the diagnosis and

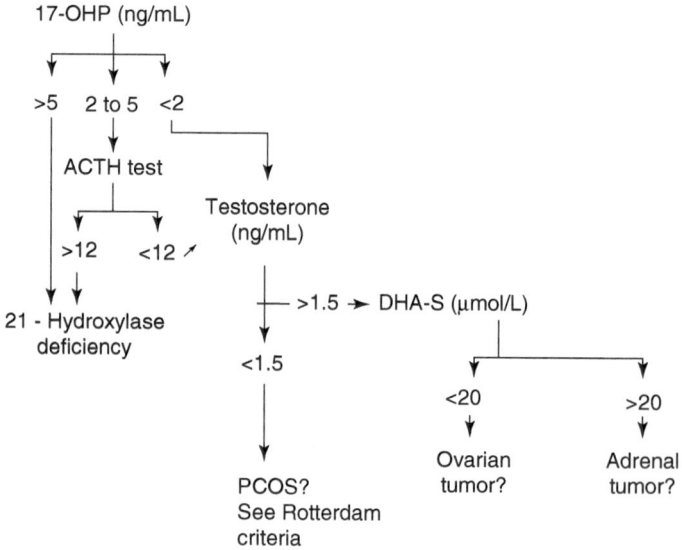

Figure 3.2 Hyperandrogenism assessment flowchart [19]

identifying severe alleles that may increase the risk of CAH in the offspring of NCAH patients [30].

A serum testosterone level >200 ng/dL is highly suggestive of an adrenal or ovarian tumor. If serum testosterone is elevated despite a normal DHEAS level, an ovarian source is more likely. If a DHEAS level >700 mcg/dL is present despite a normal serum testosterone level, an adrenal source should be suspected as the cause of hirsutism [12].

If an adrenal or ovarian tumor is suspected, adrenal or ovarian ultrasound scan/computed tomography is immediately indicated.

Mildly elevated serum testosterone and DHEAS are often present in functional ovarian hyperandrogenism (FOH) and late-onset congenital adrenal hyperplasia (CAH).

A very recent study has revealed that PCOS patients with co-elevation of androstenedione and testosterone have impaired indices of insulin sensitivity compared with those with normal androgens or milder hyperandrogenemia [31].

If PCOS is suspected, it is not useful to search an elevated serum LH level and/or an exaggerated LH response to the GnRH test and/or an elevated LH/FSH ratio, because the sensitivity of these tests are low and not recommended by the Rotterdam Consensus [19]; instead, a metabolic assessment is indicated.

The most accurate method to diagnose insulin resistance is the OGTT (oral glucose tolerance test) after 75 g glucose challenge [32]. Normal values are the following:

Glycemia:

- Fasting, 70–100 mg/dL.
- 60 min after glucose administration, <180 mg/dL.
- 120 min after glucose administration, <140 mg/dL.

Impaired glucose tolerance (IGT) is defined when glucose level is >140 mg/dL 2 h after-glucose load, but <200 mg/dL. Diabetes is defined when glycemia is >200 mg/dL 2 h-after-glucose load.

Insulinemia:

- Fasting, <10 mUI/mL.
- 60 min after glucose administration, <80 mUI/mL.
- 120 min after glucose administration, <20 mUI/mL.

Of course, the majority of PCOS patients are not diabetic yet, but only insulin-resistant; insulin resistance is defined when insulin value 1 h after OGTT is >80 mUI/mL and/or its level is not very close to the fasting insulin value after 2 h post glucose administration [26].

It has been suggested that an OGTT should be performed every 2 years for those with normal glucose tolerance and annually if IFG or IGT is present [33].

Dyslipidemia is common in PCOS and is present in up to 70% of subjects [33, 34].

The AE-PCOS Society consensus statement [33] recommends a complete lipid and hepatic profile in all patients with PCOS. Pathological values are the following:

- Total cholesterol >200 mg/dL.
- LDL cholesterol >130 mg/dL.
- HDL cholesterol <50 mg/dL.
- Triglycerides >150 mg/dL.
- AST >30 U/L.
- ALT >35 U/L.
- γ-GT >38 U/L.

From a clinical-metabolic point of view, physician should verify the presence of hypertension or clinical signs of hyper-insulinemia such as *acanthosis nigricans (AN)*.

AN is a skin lesion appearing as a thickened, velvety brown streaking to a leathery, verrucous, papillomatous change. It usually occurs on the neck or in skin folds. Microscopically, AN is characterized by an increased number of melanocytes, with papillary hypertrophy and hyperkeratosis [35]. Benign acanthosis nigricans usually correlates to insulin resistance or obesity [36, 37].

References

1. Lizneva D, Gavrilova-Jordan L, Walker W, et al. Androgen excess: investigation and management. Best Pract Res Clin Obstet Gynec. 2016;37:98–118.

2. Redmond GP, Bergfeld WF. Diagnostic approach to androgen disorders in women: acne, hirsutism, and alopecia. Cleve Clin J Med. 1990;57:423–7.

3. Uno H. Biology of hair growth. Semin Reprod Endocrinol. 1986;4:131–41.

4. Wendelin DS, Pope DN, Mallory SB. Hypertrichosis. J Am Acad Dermatol. 2003;48:161–79.

5. Al-Nuaimi Y, Baier G, Watson REB, et al. The cycling hair follicle as an ideal systems biology research model. Exp Dermatol. 2010;19:707–13.

6. Burger HG. Androgen production in women. Fertil Steril. 2002;77:S3–5.

7. Alonso L, Fuchs E. The hair cycle. J Cell Sci. 2006;119(Pt 3):391–3.

8. Azziz R, Carmina E, Sawaya ME. Idiopathic hirsutism. Endocr Rev. 2000;21(4):347–62.

9. Rosenfield RL. Hirsutism and the variable response of the pilosebaceous unit to androgen. J Investig Dermatol Symp Proc. 2005;10(3):205–8.

10. Rotaru M, Totoianu IG, Sin AI, et al. Study regarding the microscopic aspects of pilo-sebaceous units after antiandrogen treatment in hirsute women. Romanian J Morphol Embryol. 2015;56(1):63–9.

11. Escobar-Morreale HF, Carmina E, Dewailly D, et al. Epidemiology, diagnosis and management of hirsutism: a consensus statement by the androgen excess and polycystic ovary syndrome society. Hum Reprod Update. 2012;18:146–70.

12. Brodell LA, Mercurio MG. Hirsutism: diagnosis and management. Gend Med. 2010;7(2):79–87.

13. Yildiz BO, Bolour S, Woods K, et al. Visually scoring hirsutism. Hum Reprod Update. 2010;16(1):51–64.

14. McKenna TJ, Miller RB, Liddle GW. Plasma pregnenolone and 17-OH pregnenolone in patients with adrenal tumors, ACTH excess, or idiopathic hirsutism. J Clin Endocrinol Metab. 1977;44:231–6.

15. Rittmaster RS, Thompson DL. Effect of leuprolide and dexamethasone on hair growth and hormone levels in hirsute women: the relative importance of the ovary and the adrenal in the pathogenesis of hirsutism. J Clin Endocrinol Metab. 1990;70:1096–102.

16. Jahanfar S, Eden JA. Idiopathic hirsutism or polycystic ovary syndrome? Aust N Z J Obstet Gynaecol. 1993;33:414–6.

17. Azziz R, Waggoner WT, Ochoa T. Idiopathic hirsutism: an uncommon cause of hirsutism in Alabama. Fertil Steril. 1998;70:274–8.
18. Kashar-Miller M, Azziz R. Heritability and the risk of developing androgen excess. J Steroid Biochem Mol Biol. 1999;69:261–8.
19. Catteau-Jonard S, Cortet Rudelli C, et al. Hyperandrogenism in adolescent girls. Endocrin Dev. 2012;22:181–93.
20. Zouboulis CC. Acne and sebaceous gland function. Clin Dermatol. 2004;22:360–6.
21. Zouboulis CC, Degitz K. Androgen action on human skin — from basic research to clinical significance. Exp Dermatol. 2004;13(Suppl 4):5–10.
22. Makrantonaki E, Ganceviciene R, Zouboulis C. An update on the role of the sebaceous gland in the pathogenesis of acne. Dermatoendocrinol. 2011;3:41–9.
23. Adityan B, Kumari R, Thappa DM. Scoring systems in acne vulgaris. Indian J Dermatol Venereol Leprol. 2009;75:323–6.
24. Witkowsky JA, Parish LC. The assessment of acne: an evaluation of grading and lesion counting in the measurement of acne. Clin Dermatol. 2004;22:394–7.
25. Doshi A, Zaheer A, Stiller MJ. A comparison of current acne grading systems and proposal of a novel system. Int J Dermatol. 1997;36:416–8.
26. Stracquadanio M, Ciotta L. Metabolic aspects of PCOS. 2015. ISBN: 978-3-319-16759-6.
27. Olsen EA. Current and novel methods for assessing efficacy of hair growth promoters in pattern hair loss. J Am Acad Dermatol. 2003;48(2):253–62.
28. Rosenfield RL. Puberty and its disorders in girls. Endocrinol Metab Clin North Am. 1991;20:15–42.
29. Goodarzi MO, Dumesic DA, Chazenbalk G, Azziz R. Polycystic ovary syndrome: etiology, pathogenesis and diagnosis. Nat Rev Endocrinol. 2011;7:219–31.
30. Carmina E, Dewailly D, Escobar-Morreale H, et al. Non-classic congenital adrenal hyperplasia due to 21-hydroxylase deficiency revisited: an update with a special focus on adolescent and adult women. Hum Reprod Update. 2017;23:580–99.
31. O'Reilly MW, et al. Hyperandrogenemia predicts metabolic phenotype in polycystic ovary syndrome: the utility of serum androstenedione. J Clin Endocrinol Metab. 2014;99(3):1027–36.
32. Palmert MR, Gordon CM, Kartashov AI, et al. Screening for abnormal glucose tolerance in adolescents with polycystic ovary syndrome. J Clin Endocrinol Metab. 2002;87(3):1017–23.

33. Wild RA, Carmina E, Diamanti KE, et al. Assessment of cardiovascular risk and prevention of cardiovascular disease in women with the polycystic ovary syndrome: a consensus statement by the Androgen Excess and Polycystic Ovary Syndrome (AE-PCOS) Society. J Clin Endocrinol Metab. 2010;95:2039–49.
34. Rizzo M, Longo RA, Guastella E. Assessing cardiovascular risk in Mediterranean women with polycystic ovary syndrome. J Endocrinol Investig. 2011;34:422–6.
35. Dong Z, Huang J, et al. Associations of acanthosis nigricans with metabolic abnormalities in polycystic ovary syndrome women with normal body mass index. J Dermatol. 2013;40:188–92.
36. Stoddart ML, Blevins KS, Lee ET, et al. Association of acanthosis nigricans with hyperinsulinemia compared with other selected risk factors for type 2 diabetes in Cherokee Indians: the Cherokee Diabetes Study. Diabetes Care. 2002;25:1009–14.
37. Kahn CR, Flier JS, Bar RS, et al. The syndromes of insulin resistance and acanthosis nigricans insulin-receptor disorders in man. N Engl J Med. 1976;294:739–45.

Chapter 4
Treatments

4.1 Oral Contraceptives (OCs)

4.1.1 Mechanisms of Action

Oral contraceptive pills (OCPs) are considered the first-line pharmacological therapy for hyperandrogenic PCOS patients who are not trying to conceive [1, 2].

OCPs work as anti-androgens through various mechanisms [3]:

1. Estrogen increases hepatic production of sex hormone-binding globulin (SHBG), in order to reduce circulating free testosterone levels [4].
2. Progestin suppression of luteinizing hormone (LH) secretion decreases ovarian androgen production [5].
3. Progestins compete to differing extents for 5α-reductase and the androgen receptor [2, 6, 7].

Ethnicity does not influence the effects of OCPs, because patterns of increase and decrease of serum androgens and SHBG are similar regardless of race [8].

© Springer Nature Switzerland AG 2020   35
M. Stracquadanio, *Managing Women's Hyperandrogenism*,
https://doi.org/10.1007/978-3-030-29223-2_4

The ideal contraceptive for PCOS women should [9]:

- Limit antral follicle development and reduce the quantity of androgens.
- Neutralize the effect of androgens on pilosebaceous units at peripheral level.
- Restore the balance between estrogens and progesterone in the endometrium, ensuring control of the menstrual cycle.

4.1.2 Estrogens and Progestins: Making the Right Choice

Every anti-androgenic OCP contains estradiol and a synthetic progestin.

Estradiol valerate (EV2) is immediately cleaved to estradiol after oral intake: thus, the circulating molecule reaching the estrogen receptors is the natural 17β-estradiol [10].

However, the most commonly used estradiol is ethinyl estradiol (EE): it is more potent than estradiol, due to the presence of the 17-α-ethinyl group; after oral administration, EE undergoes glucuronidation and sulfation by specific enzyme [11].

The bioavailability of oral EE ranges from 38% to 48%, due to a high first-pass metabolism [12].

The dose of EE in OCPs varies from 15 μg in the latest pills to 50 μg of very old formulations [5].

The possibility that an ovarian follicle grows up to the size of a dominant follicle is greater with a daily dose of 20 μg in comparison to a dose of 30 μg [13]. Residual follicular activity is responsible not only for ovarian estradiol synthesis but also for androgen production [1, 14].

Studies have revealed that at least 50 μg of ethinyl estradiol is required for a beneficial response on hyperandrogenic PCOS patients when administered alone and not in combined OCP; because the risk of deep venous thrombosis (DVT) from estrogen is dose-dependent, the use of estrogens at these high doses is not strongly recommended [5, 15].

Thus, it is imperative to use formulation containing low dose of estrogens plus progestins, which are used to block the proliferation action of estrogens on endometrial growth [5].

Actually, in PCOS treatment protocols, it is recommended to use an anti-androgenic progestin rather than a low-androgenic progestin [16] (Table 4.1): indeed, it was shown that after 12 months of therapy, OCPs containing anti-androgenic pills show much stronger positive effects on PCOS symptoms compared to pills with low-androgenic progestin, such as desogestrel [17].

OCP composition (in terms of monophasic, biphasic, or triphasic) does not influence the mechanism through which EP improves PCOS hyperandrogenism [1]. Monophasic OCP should be the first choice due to the easier transition to continuous use. Indeed, during the 7-day pill-free interval, an increase in gonadotropin levels stimulates the ovarian

TABLE 4.1 Type and activity of progestins

Activity	Progestin	Derived from
Pure progestin activity	Nomegestrol acetate	Progesterone
Progestin activity + anti-androgenic activity	Chlormadinone acetate	Progesterone
	Cyproterone acetate	
	Dienogest	Testosterone
Progestin activity + low glucocorticoid activity	Medroxyprogesterone acetate	Progesterone
Progestin activity + anti-androgenic activity + anti-aldosterone activity	Drospirenone	Spironolactone
Residual androgenic activity	Levonorgestrel	Testosterone
	Desogestrel	
	Etonogestrel	
	Gestodene	

synthesis of androgens: for this reason, testosterone levels are significantly lower during the continuous regimen in comparison to the cyclic one, with an 86% increase in testosterone after 7 days of placebo [18].

4.1.3   Cyproterone Acetate (CPA)

It is a 17-hydroxyprogesterone derivative that inhibits the activity of 5α-reductase, competing with dihydrotestosterone (DHT) for androgen receptor binding.

It also acts by decreasing testosterone and androstenedione production through a negative feedback on the hypothalamic-pituitary axis and inhibiting LH secretion [19].

The formulation CPA 2 mg/EE 35 μg is used in Europe and Canada, but it is not approved by the Food and Drug Administration (FDA) for use in the United States [3]; it significantly improves hirsutism in PCOS patients [20, 21].

Moreover, administration of cyproterone acetate only at relatively high daily doses of 50–100 mg for 10 days of every month has been associated with a 75% improvement of acne (available only in Europe and in Canada) [15].

As a non-OCP medication, CPA is given from the first until the tenth day of the menstrual cycle (day 1 is commonly the first day of menstruation) [22].

After CPA treatment the hair changes usually are the infringement of the hair follicle development in incipient stages of the sheath and matrix formation and the formation of air areas inside the medulla. The diameter of the hair follicle was reduced to 0.03 mm, sebaceous elements were attenuated, and the arrector pili muscles were fragmented in a way that deterred them from contributing to the verticalization of hair follicles [23, 24].

4.1.4   Chlormadinone Acetate (CMA)

It is a 17-acetoxyprogesterone derivative molecule, with a strong affinity for the progesterone receptors [25, 26]. CMA exerts a low glucocorticoid activity [21, 27] and a potent anti-androgenic effect [27–30], by competition with endogenous androgens at target receptors in skin and hair and by inhibition of 5α-reductase type 1. CMA does not bind to SHBG [31], allowing the EP formulation containing EE + CMA to cause a significant reduction in androgen bioavailability [32].

This EP association seems to be effective in the treatment of moderate acne and seborrhea [33]: indeed CMA reduces the activity of skin 5α-reductase, the enzyme converting testosterone to the more potent 5α-dihydrotestosterone [30].

4.1.5 Drospirenone (DRSP)

It explicates anti-androgenic and mineralocorticoid properties: in fact, it derives from 17α-spironolactone and thus has anti-androgenic activity similar to that of spironolactone [34].

Drospirenone has a bioavailability of 76% with approximately 20% excreted through the feces and 45% through the renal system; its half-life is 30 h [35].

Drospirenone treats hyperandrogenism by multiple effects:

– Reduction of ovarian steroid production.
– Blockage of peripheral androgen receptors in the dermis and pilosebaceous units [36].
– Decrease of adrenal androgen synthesis, through interaction with adrenal androgen receptors. There is evidence suggesting that androgens may directly affect adrenal hormonal secretion [37].

It does not adversely affect the estrogen-induced increase of SHBG levels, and it does not interfere with androgen binding to SHBG [12, 38, 39].

Drospirenone is able to induce sodium excretion and a compensatory increase in renin secretion, plasma renin activity, angiotensin II, and plasma aldosterone, minimizing the estrogen-related fluid retention [40].

Thus, because it is an aldosterone antagonist, drospirenone exerts a diuretic effect that can reduce premenstrual symptoms (abdominal bloating and breast tenderness) [40–43] and blood pressure rise [44].

Moreover, it has been shown that drospirenone-containing OCPs do not cause any increase in BMI; thus they are a good option for treatment of obese PCOS patients [44]. Drospirenone is more likely than other progestins to favor rather than inhibit the loss of weight, and it may provide an advantage in terms of patient's compliance [45].

FDA approves the formulation drospirenone 3 mg/EE 20 μg for the treatment of acne, but not for hirsutism therapy [3].

However, the literature data support the efficacy of drospirenone/EE 30 μg for the first-line hirsutism treatment [21, 36, 44]. Trials show an initial beneficial effect on hirsutism after 6 months of therapy, and then it is indicated to change regimen [46, 47].

4.1.6   Dienogest (DNG)

Dienogest is chemically described as (17β)-17-hydroxy-3-oxo-19-norpregna-4,9-diene-21-nitrile, and it is structurally related to the norethindrone family, but acts as an anti-androgen [48]: indeed, it is designed to specifically bind to progesterone receptor [49].

DNG may also have a direct action on 5α-reductase, so its use is particularly effective in the treatment of acne and seborrhea [50, 51].

The association E2V/DNG could be recommended in PCOS women with IR or who are overweight [9] because its effects on prothrombin, D-dimer, HDL, LDL insulin, and carbohydrate metabolism are more favorable [52].

4.1.7   Side Effects and Contraindications of EP

EPs are contraindicated in smokers, patients suffering from migraines, women with history of stroke or hypertension, and patients with personal or family history of thromboembolism, liver disease, and diabetes [3] (Table 4.2).

TABLE 4.2 Contraindications for OCPs [53]

Contraindications for hormonal therapy
– Pregnancy
– Breastfeeding
– <6 months post-partum
– History of stroke
– History of venous thromboembolism
– History of myocardial infarction
– Smoking of any amount and above 35 years old
– Uncontrolled hypertension
– History of migraine with focal symptoms/aura
– History of migraine and age above 35 years
– Current or past history of breast cancer
– Hypercholesterolemia
– Diabetes and age above 35 years
– End-organ damage (liver, kidney)
– Viral hepatitis or cirrhosis
– Liver tumor (any type)

4.1.8   Cardiovascular Risk

Patients should be counseled that the risk factors for cardio-vascular events include smoking (any amount), hypertension, and diabetes [53].

According to the World Health Organization (WHO), the use of estro-progestins increases the cardiovascular risk only in women who already have a recognized predisposition to it [54].

In women with established hypertension, two studies reported a further increase in blood pressure, but this result was not found to be conclusive [55].

Ethinyl estradiol, because of its greater potency compared with estradiol, exacerbates the production of hepatic angio-tensinogen, which causes an elevation of arterial pressure via the renin-angiotensin-aldosterone system [56].

Hypertension and OCP may act synergistically to increase the risk of myocardial infarction and stroke, but the evidence is unsatisfying: in fact, the estimated incidence of cardiovascular events is low even in hypertensive women who take EPs (3 events per 10.000 woman-years between 20 and 40 years of age) [55, 57].

According to the WHO guidelines, the use of EP is contraindicated in hypertensive women, regardless of the administration route, being considered of category 3 (the risks exceed the benefits) and 4 (the risks make it unacceptable for use) [58].

There are few suggestions that women with PCOS, without any other apparent disease, may have an increased risk of cardiovascular pathologies compared to normal women of similar age and BMI [45, 59].

The mechanisms explaining how OCPs cause excessive local activation of coagulation, causing thrombus growth, are not completely clear [60]. Recently, it has been suggested that the activation of the CD40/CD40L pathway may enhance pro-coagulant activity and thrombus formation. sCD40 ligation on cells of the vascular wall promotes mononuclear cell recruitment [61]; sCD40L and CD40 participate in the initial event in atherothrombosis, leading to the activation of several pro-inflammatory, pro-atherosclerotic, and coagulation mediators [62].

A recent Turkish study demonstrated that OCP increased circulating sCD40L concentrations [60].

A careful family history of thromboembolic events must be obtained and, when in doubt, factor V Leiden deficiency should be ruled out [63].

Hyper-homocysteinemia (hyper-Hcy) is considered an independent risk factor for cardiovascular diseases [45]. Indeed, elevated plasma Hcy levels are associated with an increased risk of atherosclerotic coronary, cerebral, and peripheral vascular disease [64]. It was also observed that hyper-Hcy is present in PCOS women, suggesting that an alteration in Hcy metabolism may be implicated in the increased risk of cardiovascular disease in this kind of patients [45].

Moreover, other studies showed a significant increase in homocysteine levels during and after OCP treatment [65–67].

Thus, Hcy serum dosage might be useful to select patients at risk of cardiovascular disease. However, there are currently no routine follow-up screening guidelines for OC prescription [47].

The increased risk of venous thromboembolism (VTE) depends on the dose of EE and the type of progestin included in the OCP.

Ethinyl estradiol induces significant changes in the coagulation system leading to an increase in thrombin generation. It has been reported that EE causes an enhancement in coagulation factors (fibrinogen and factors VII, VIII, IX, X, XII, and XIII) and a reduction in the natural inhibitors of coagulation (protein S and antithrombin), producing a mild pro-coagulant effect [68, 69].

The progestogens with a greater anti-androgen effect present in OCPs seem to increase the risk of thromboembolic events [70].

Indeed, levonorgestrel increases VTE risk 3.6-fold, gestodene 5.6-fold, desogestrel 7.3-fold, CPA 6.8-fold, and drospirenone 6.3-fold, compared to non-OC users [71].

Moreover, it is well known that VTE risk increases in relation to EE dosage, especially with EE >50 µg [72]. To increase the safety and tolerability of the contraceptive pills, over the years the included dose of ethinyl estradiol has been reduced to 20–35 µg [73].

However, VTE often occurs, during the first year of treatment, in patients >35 years old with at least one risk factor for thrombotic disease [71, 74–76].

Thus, in PCOS patients with increased cardiovascular risk factors, it is essential to evaluate the risk-benefit ratio [3].

PCOS is also linked to chronic inflammation and endothelial dysfunction [77], which are characterized by elevated serum adhesion molecules [78]: in fact, PCOS women show increased ICAM-1 [79–82] and MCP-1 concentrations [83–86].

Intercellular adhesion molecule-1 (ICAM-1) is expressed on the surface of the endothelium cells, smooth muscle cells, macrophages, and activated lymphocytes and plays an important role in the adhesion of circulating leukocytes to the blood vessel wall and trans-endothelial migration to vascular intima [87, 88].

Some evidence suggests that OCP use may worsen sub-inflammation and consequent risk of cardiovascular disease [89, 90]. However, data in literature are controversial: OCP use may increase [91], or decrease [92, 93], or have no effect on ICAM-1 [94].

Matrix metallo-proteinases (MMPs) are proteolytic enzymes that degrade extracellular collagen and participate in vascular remodeling [95]: thus, they are involved in atherosclerosis process. Women with PCOS have imbalances in circulating MMPs, probably due to their hyperandrogenemia [96]. In fact, a recent study showed that an anti-androgenic OCP reduced plasma concentrations of MMP-2 in women with PCOS [95].

Moreover, high-sensitivity C-reactive protein (hsCRP) is a marker for the evaluation of cardiovascular risk and inflammatory pathway [97]; some studies reported that its levels are increased in PCOS women [98, 99] and the use of OCPs might result in elevated hsCRP levels [100–102].

These mechanisms are not well known; the liver is the main origin of CRP synthesis, which is stimulated by OCPs, and therefore this increase may be attributed to increased hepatic synthesis [100, 101, 103].

A very recent study proved that patients taking EE/CMA showed a significant increase in the hsCRP levels when compared with PCOS women assuming EE/DRSP pill at 6, 12, and 24 months [104].

Even follistatin, a carrier protein of the TGF-β (transforming growth factor-β) superfamily, has a role in the modulation of the inflammatory reaction and in the occurrence of atherosclerosis [105, 106], and it was found to be increased in obese women with PCOS after OCP treatment, and it could be considered an indicator of an increased risk of future cardiovascular disease [101].

Endothelial dysfunction presents early in the atherosclerotic process long before structural vascular lesions occur [107]. A recent study showed that CIMT (carotid intima-media thickness), an indicator of early atherosclerosis, and FMD (brachial artery flow-mediated dilatation), a finding of endothelial dysfunction, seem to be deteriorated after 6-month follow-up of PCOS patients who were taking OCPs [108]. Conversely, a recent study showed that EP administration improves FMD parameter in young non-obese PCOS patients [108], stating that androgens' decrease may contribute to improved endothelial function in PCOS women via ameliorating of insulin resistance that is associated with endothelial dysfunction [109].

Because smoking deteriorates endothelial function and amplifies the blood coagulation abnormalities, smoking cessation should be aggressively promoted in PCOS patients [110].

4.1.9 Breast Cancer Risk

OCP use has also been associated with elevated premenopausal breast cancer risk [111, 112]. However, prior studies assessing the possible association between PCOS and breast cancer report conflicting results, including increased risk [113], decreased risk [114], and null results [114–116].

The exact mechanism of OCP contribution to carcinogenesis is not completely clear, but there are several options. Estrogens and progestogens induce breast cell proliferation, particularly when both hormones are present [117]. In general, the breasts of women taking the combined OCP are exposed to the combined proliferative effects of estrogen and progestogens for longer per cycle than those not taking the OCP, possibly increasing the risk of DNA damage and neoplastic transformation [118].

One of the first meta-analyses conducted in 1996 showed that women on OCP were found to have an increased relative risk of 1.24 of developing breast cancer, with risk declining up to 10 years following cessation of OCP; after 10 years of cessation of OCP, there was no significant increase in the relative risk of breast cancer. Current or past history of breast cancer is currently a contraindication for OCP use [53].

4.1.10   Metabolic Effects of EP

The possibility that OCPs might alter the lipid profile and glucose tolerance should be considered before prescribing these drugs to PCOS patients, since they are more disposed to develop insulin resistance, metabolic syndrome, and diabetes mellitus [119–121].

4.1.11   Carbohydrate Metabolism

EP may increase insulin resistance [2, 122] but data in literature are heterogeneous [44, 123]. The estrogen and progestin components of OCPs could independently influence carbohydrate metabolism [5].

It was shown that ethinyl estradiol increases the glucose response in an oral glucose tolerance test (OGTT) causing insulin resistance [124]; using a reduced dose of ethinyl estradiol (from 50 to 20 μg) could decrease the severity of hyperinsulinemia. OCPs containing low dose of EE exert no significant effects on carbohydrate metabolism in nondiabetic women [125].

However some authors consider the progestin agent as primarily responsible for this metabolic effect [5, 124, 126]: the negative effects of the progestins are related to their intrinsic androgenicity [127].

For these reasons, caution should be taken when prescribing EP to PCOS patients who are obese, are insulin-resistant, or have a family history of diabetes [5].

Nader and Diamanti-Kandarakis devised four groups (or quartiles) of PCOS patients according to an arbitrary scale of insulin sensitivity [128]:

  – *Quartile 1: these PCOS patients have near-normal genetic insulin sensitivity; they are thin, and their only adverse factor is their androgenicity. Treatment with OCP may lead to improvement in carbohydrate metabolism (lowering of androgens improves glucose tolerance).*

- *Quartile 2: these patients have near-normal or mildly impaired genetic insulin sensitivity. They may be of normal weight or mildly overweight. Their androgenicity is also an adverse factor. Treatment with OCP may show now change in carbohydrate metabolism (as the potential impairment of glucose tolerance by the OCP is offset by the androgen-lowering effect of the pill).*
- *Quartile 3: these women may have a moderate impaired genetic insulin sensitivity. They may be moderately overweight. Other adverse factors could include their androgenicity, puberty, or the use of OCP. The outcome with OCP treatment may be deterioration in carbohydrate metabolism (impairment of glucose tolerance by the OCP may be greater than the benefit of the androgen-lowering effect of the pill).*
- *Quartile 4: these individuals have severely impaired genetic insulin sensitivity. They may be severely obese. Other adverse factors include their androgenicity, puberty, or the use of an androgenic OCP. The outcome of OCP treatment may possibly be the development of frank diabetes.*

It is possible that obesity amplifies EP adverse effects on glucose tolerance [129]; however, the results of a very recent study showed that in obese PCOS women who were already strongly insulin-resistant at baseline, OCPs did not further aggravate this insulin resistance; only control women had a significant increase in fasting insulin and worsening of insulin sensitivity after 3 months of OC when compared to baseline. However, even after this worsening of insulin sensitivity with OCPs, control women were still more insulin-sensitive compared to PCOS women [129].

Vaginal ring containing etonogestrel (a low-androgenic progestin) appears to be better for this kind of women because of its lower effect on insulin resistance. The latter may be due to its controlled steady-state release of hormones and to a smaller systemic hormone dose exposure [130].

Conversely, few studies have shown that OCPs containing EE 20 μg or 30 μg + drospirenone 3 mg do not cause any worsening of glucose tolerance or insulin resistance even after 12 months of treatment [8, 44, 73, 131, 132].

In fact, it has been hypothesized that aldosterone induces insulin resistance [133, 134], and therefore the anti-mineralocorticoid effect of drospirenone also has a beneficial effect on insulin sensitivity [135].

4.1.12   Lipid Profile

EP may increase triglycerides, and so should be avoided in women with hypertriglyceridemia [70, 136, 137].

Conversely, Escobar-Morreale et al. reported that triglycerides remained unchanged in adult hirsute women who were treated by an OCP containing desogestrel [138].

However, a past NIH consensus shows that the atherosclerotic risk is not increased by an estrogen-induced rise in triglyceride levels if the level of high-density lipoprotein (HDL) cholesterol remains high and the level of low-density lipoprotein (LDL) cholesterol is not increased [73, 139, 140].

Literature is inconsistent in stating unanimously that OCPs cause a rise in LDL cholesterol: some authors reported an increase [141–144], while others did not observe any change in LDL levels [136].

A very recent study proved that patients taking EE/CMA showed a significant increase in the total cholesterol level when compared with PCOS women assuming EE/DRSP pill at 6, 12, and 24 months [104].

It is necessary to point out that hyperinsulinemic PCOS women at baseline show reduced HDL cholesterol and increased total cholesterol, LDL cholesterol, and triglyceride serum levels when compared with healthy controls [142–144]: thus, it is important to first treat insulin resistance and then to evaluate the administration of OCPs.

4.1.13 Adiponectin Levels

Adiponectin presents anti-inflammatory and insulin-sensitizing effects [132], and its levels are decreased in PCOS patients: this abnormality is independent from the grade of obesity, being present even in lean women with this syndrome [108, 145].

A Spanish study demonstrated that the administration of an anti-androgenic OCP increases adiponectin secretion, as a result of the amelioration of androgen excess. Thus, this result supports the hypothesis that hyperandrogenemia has a direct inhibitory effect on adiponectin secretion by adipocytes [8].

4.1.14 Bone Mineral Density (BMD)

Contraceptives may also positively influence skeletal homeostasis through estradiol inhibiting bone reabsorption [146] and promoting BMD maintenance. Longitudinal general population studies also report inverse association between contraceptive use and fracture risk [147]. However, the association of contraceptive use with BMD in PCOS has not been fully investigated and understood [148].

In fact, some studies report higher BMD in PCOS [149] probably because testosterone inhibits bone reabsorption in vivo [146] or through peripheral conversion to 17β-estradiol and estrone [150]. It is possible that the effects of OCPs on BMD may be worsened in the hyperandrogenic state of PCOS, because EP reduces bioavailable androgens [148].

4.2 Anti-Androgen Drugs

4.2.1 Making the Right Choice: Side Effects and Contraindications

Spironolactone

It is an aldosterone antagonist acting through a dose-dependent mechanism of action. Spironolactone has multiple anti-androgenic effects [46, 151–153]:

- Inhibition of ovarian and adrenal androgen production.
- Competitive blockage of the skin androgen receptor.
- Elevation of SHBG levels.
- Increased testosterone clearance.
- Inhibition of 5α-reductase.

A dose of spironolactone is equivalent to CPA 1 mg and drospirenone 3 mg [154].

The appropriate initial dose for lean PCOS women is 100 mg daily, but higher doses are necessary for women with severe hirsutism or obesity [4, 151].

No serious complications were reported with the administration of spironolactone; rare side effects include hyperkalemia (increased if there is a concomitant liver or kidney disease) [155], fatigue, breast tenderness, and headaches.

A recent study showed no increased risk of breast cancer with spironolactone [156].

It is recommended to check the baseline potassium level, repeated after 1 month and after dose increases. OC should be prescribed with spironolactone, if it is possible, to avoid teratogenicity, feminization of a male fetus, and menstrual irregularities [3]: indeed the major side effect encountered after spironolactone treatment is polymenorrhea, which can be observed in 50% of cases [157].

Spironolactone should be avoided with angiotensin-converting enzyme (ACE) inhibitors and high dose of non-steroidal anti-inflammatory drugs [3].

A starting dose of 25 mg/day should be increased over several weeks to minimize side effects [5].

A recent study showed an improvement in endothelial function with spironolactone treatment, which could be in part a consequence of aldosterone antagonism [158] and might be due to its androgenic effects too [159]. In fact, endothelial dysfunction in PCOS patients was found to be associated also to androgens [107, 160–162]. Androgen receptors are present on the vessel wall [163], and testosterone was shown to worsen endothelial function [164].

4.2.2 Finasteride

It is a progesterone derivative that blocks the conversion of testosterone to dihydrotestosterone (DHT) inhibiting 5α-reductase [165].

The fall in serum DHT is accompanied by a reduction in metabolites of DHT such as 3α-diol G and by a rise in plasma testosterone concentrations [166].

It was released in 1992 for the treatment of prostatic disorders [151, 167]; thus its use in PCOS treatment is off-label. The most used dose is 5 mg per day, even if studies indicate equal efficacy with 2.5 mg per day [168].

Common side effects are dry skin, libido reduction, headache, and gastrointestinal disorders [169–172].

Recently, it was shown that a low-dose (2.5 mg) administration of finasteride, given every 3 days, is effective in reducing hirsutism, with the advantage to minimize both side effects and treatment costs [173].

It could be hepatotoxic and it is unsafe during pregnancy (possible interference with the normal development of a male fetus): for these reasons it is important to recommend:

- Liver enzyme blood test every 3 months.
- Contemporaneous contraception method [3].

Finasteride is particularly used for the treatment of hirsutism or defluvium (very high affinity for 5α-reductase isoenzyme 2) [173], while it is not recommended for the cure of acne because its affinity for the type I isoenzyme of 5α-reductase (which is involved in the formation of acne) is very low [15, 174].

4.2.3 Flutamide

It is a very potent non-steroidal androgen antagonist used in prostate cancer treatment.

Its mechanisms of action include [175, 176]:

- Blockage of the androgen receptor (without any interactions with glucocorticoid, progesterone, or estrogen receptors).

- Interference with cellular uptake of testosterone and DHT.
- Increased androgen metabolism to inactive compounds.
- Possible direct inhibition of adrenal androgen production [177].

Flutamide has no progestogenic or anti-gonadotropin action, and thus it does not alter the mechanism of ovulation [178] nor cause menstrual irregularity [157].

Even better, a recent study demonstrated that the treatment with flutamide induces improvement of menstrual cyclicity and ovulatory status in PCOS patients by a series of events [179]:

- The evident decrease of androgen secretion and the increase of estrogen production that help to normalize the altered androgen-to-estrogen ratio in the ovary [180].
- The reduction of LH secretion and the consequent rebalancing of the compromised gonadotropin secretion, which contribute to restore the sensitivity of the GnRH pulse generator to feedback inhibition by sexual steroids, at hypothalamic level [181].

After oral administration, flutamide is split into numerous plasma metabolites, among which 2-hydroxyflutamide is responsible for the drug's anti-androgenic activity [182].

The suggested dose is 250 mg daily [176], but lower doses seem to have fairly the same effects with fewer side effects [175, 183].

Decreases in androstenedione [184–186], testosterone [186, 187], and DHEAS [184–188] levels have been reported.

The metabolic effects of flutamide in PCOS are different [177]:

- No change [184] or improvements in insulin sensitivity [187, 189].
- Decreases in triglycerides and LDL cholesterol levels have been found in obese and lean PCOS hyperandrogenic women [186, 189].
- Increase in HDL cholesterol levels [189].
- Increased leptin levels: testosterone inhibits lipid uptake and lipoprotein lipase activity in adipocytes, with a

decreased production of leptin. Since flutamide binds to androgen receptors and blocks their actions, it also causes an increase in leptin levels [190].

Flutamide treatment can be complicated by skin dryness, gastrointestinal discomfort, breast tenderness [157], hot flashes, and decreased libido [53].

It might be hepatotoxic, and usually this side effect occurs within 3 months of therapy [191, 192]. It has been reported that ALT levels in patients taking flutamide were associated with past history of liver disorders [193]. The mechanism of hepatotoxicity is not completely clear, but it is dose-dependent; probably it is due to biotransformation of flutamide into electrophilic metabolites by cytochrome P450s (CYPs) [194]: the reactive metabolites bind to microsomal proteins, leading to toxic or immune hepatitis in patients [193].

Thus, it is recommended to monitor AST and ALT blood levels every 3 months during treatment with flutamide for at least 1 year [193].

Flutamide is also considered unsafe during pregnancy (possible interference with the normal development of a male fetus); thus a contemporaneous contraception method must be advised [3].

Flutamide 250 mg daily may be more effective than finasteride in treating hirsutism in PCOS women [170, 193, 195].

Moreover, one of the first randomized controlled trials showed that combination of flutamide/OCP seems to improve acne by 80%, while spironolactone/OC improves acne by only 50% [196].

Flutamide is actually not approved for pediatric use, even off-label [63].

4.3   Glucocorticoids

Glucocorticoids (GCs) are traditionally used for the treatment of hyperandrogenism in women with congenital adrenal hyperplasia, but its long-term use is very controversial [197]. It aims to reduce adrenal hyperandrogenism, while the necessity for cortisol replacement is less evident. Low doses of dexamethasone are needed (0.25–0.5 mg at night), instead of hydrocortisone and prednisone that are less potent ACTH-inhibiting compounds [198]. The target is not to normalize the morning 17 OHP plasma level, since it has been shown that adrenal androgens are more sensitive to the glucocorticoid-suppressive effect than the C-21 steroids [199]. Thus, it is necessary to monitor the testosterone or androstenedione plasma levels; in case of pregnancy wish, the progesterone serum level should be monitored during the follicular phase in order to avoid anti-cervical mucus effect [198].

Treatment with glucocorticoids for NCAH should be considered only for pre- and peripubertal children who have inappropriately early onset or rapid progression of pubarche or bone age. In adolescents and young adults with NCAH, treatment is reserved for those who demonstrate important or clinically significant hyperandrogenism; ovarian androgen suppression or peripheral androgen blockade is more effective than glucocorticoids for reducing circulating androgens and their effects. Adult women with NCAH who have not conceived spontaneously and demonstrate subclinical ovulatory dysfunction may benefit from glucocorticoids or from ovulation induction [200].

4.4   Lifestyle Modifications

Women with insulin resistance should follow some useful advices for their daily diet [201]:

- Eat 5–10 different whole fresh fruits, vegetables, and legumes each day.
- Avoid a diet that consists predominantly of the food highest on the glycemic index (GI).
- Substitute foods high on the GI with foods lower on the GI: for example, eat boiled green beans (GI of 15) instead of boiled potatoes (GI of 100) with dinner.
- Increase fiber intake: fiber helps to slow the digestion of carbohydrates and improves insulin resistance. If a food high on the GI is loved, patient should take care not to consume it often and aim to eat only a small portion of

it combined with high-fiber foods that reduce the glycemic index [202, 203].

– Eat legumes to lower the high-GI foods in the meals: legumes are low on the GI and contain an impressive amount of fiber and good-quality protein, which can serve to blunt the glycemic load. Moreover, legumes contain pinitol, a relative of D-chiro-inositol, noted for improving insulin resistance [204].

– Avoid overeating foods high on the glycemic index. The GI of a food can be tempered by the quantity consumed. For example, a piece of candy might have a very high glycemic index, but eating just one little piece will not result in a high glycemic load on the body; if the patient eats two pieces of white toast, jam, brown potatoes, and a sugar- or corn syrup-sweetened fruit drink for breakfast, she is putting a high glycemic load on her body, and the blood sugar will remain high for several hours as her body works to process the large amount of high-GI foods [204].

– Evaluate the whole meat, rather than individual food items, to make sure the patient is preparing meals that will not spike her blood sugars.

Exercise reduces insulin resistance by two mechanisms. It induces a reduction in visceral fat even if it results in moderate weight loss and BMI reduction [205]. Visceral fat is more metabolically active than subcutaneous fat and central adiposity is more closely related to IR [206].

Besides, exercise increases muscle cell metabolism: it modulates the expression or the activity of proteins mediating insulin signaling in the skeletal muscles [205, 207].

It has been shown that exercise improves menstrual abnormalities and restores ovulation in obese patients with PCOS [208], and its benefit on reproductive function is greater than the benefit of low-calorie diet only [209].

Exercise exerts its beneficial effects on body composition with a 45% greater reduction in fat mass and a 60% better preservation of fat-free mass [210].

In fact, it is important to clarify that improved abdominal obesity and insulin sensitivity may occur without a total change in body weight: body composition of patients who exercise regularly may change with increased lean body mass and decreased fat mass, but no overall change in weight [211].

4.5   Insulin Sensitizers

According to the ASRM Committee of 2008, insulin-sensitizing agents should be considered in patients with impaired glucose tolerance (IGT) and PCOS [212].

Particularly, in 2010, AE-PCOS Society consensus treatment emphasized that metformin should be used in women with PCOS who have already started lifestyle treatment (diet and exercise) and do not have improvement in IGT, or in those who have normal weight but still having IGT [204].

When administered to insulin-resistant patients, these drugs act to increase target tissue responsiveness, in order to reduce hyperinsulinemia [213].

In the past, limited studies on the use of diazoxide, acarbose, and somatostatin for PCOS women were conducted; then, thiazolidinediones aroused more interest, while, to date, metformin is the most worldwide studied insulin-sensitizing agent.

To date neither in Europe nor in the United States has metformin been approved for the treatment of insulin resistance associated to PCOS: its use should be restricted to those patients with IGT [214]; however, it is largely prescribed as an "off-label" drug.

During the last two decades, some studies demonstrated that metformin inhibits androstenedione and testosterone production from theca cells through inhibition of the steroidogenic acute regulatory protein and 17α-hydroxylase expression [206].

At the ovarian level, hyper-androgenic intra-follicular pattern is improved by a decrease in IGF-I availability that has an important role in controlling granulosa cell aromatase levels [215].

Metformin is available as 500-, 850-, and 1000-mg tablets with a target dose of 1500–2550 mg/day.

Metformin has a dose-dependent absorption in humans [216], and its bioavailability is limited to 50–60% because the amount available may result from pre-systemic clearance or binding to the intestinal wall [216].

Therapeutic regimens of metformin administration are not well standardized, and its dose should probably be adjusted according to the patient's BMI and insulin resistance [217].

For example, it was demonstrated that non-obese women with PCOS respond better than obese women to metformin treatment at a dosage of 1500 mg/day for 6 months. Non-obese women, in fact, showed a statistically significant decrease in serum androgen level and fasting insulin level and also an improvement in menstrual cyclicity [218]. Moreover, it is possible that women who did not respond to metformin 1.5 g dose per day might show clinical changes if the dose is increased to 2 g [219].

Common side effects are gastrointestinal, such as diarrhea, nausea, vomiting, bloating, abdominal discomfort, flatulence, and unpleasant metallic taste in mouth.

Lactic acidosis and hypoglycemia are very rare.

To reduce these side effects, it is recommended to start metformin with a low dose (e.g., 250–500 mg/day) and then gradually increase within a period of 4–6 weeks [219].

Metformin may cause vitamin B12 malabsorption, and so every patient should be monitored for signs and symptoms of vitamin B12 deficiency: numbness, paresthesia, macroglossia, behavioral changes, and pernicious anemia [220].

Metformin prescription should be avoided in women with renal insufficiency, congestive heart failure, sepsis, or hepatic dysfunction [220].

Therefore, testing of hepatic and renal function is necessary in advance of prescription, and thereafter yearly testing is indicated.

However, it has been demonstrated that metformin use for up to 6 months does not adversely affect renal or liver function in a large sample of PCOS women, even those with mildly abnormal baseline hepatic parameters [205, 207].

Metformin determines a great improvement on the hyperandrogenism symptoms of patients with PCOS, ameliorating hyperandrogenemia, and reducing circulating insulin levels [221, 222]. Moreover, as insulin acts as an anabolic growth factor in hair [222], it is possible that the suppression of circulating insulin levels alone may be sufficient to improve the rate of terminal hair growth [219].

A 20–30% reduction of total and free testosterone, increased SHBG levels, a 30% decline of androstenedione levels, a modest decrease of FG hirsutism score, and an improvement of acanthosis nigricans were shown [223].

Poor effects on the acne score of young PCOS women were recorded [224].

Several data suggest that metformin could act on hyperandrogenism by interfering both with direct and specific mechanisms on peripheral androgen-secreting organs and with free androgen fraction-regulating systems [214]: in fact, a reduced ovarian and adrenal secretion of androgens, a reduced pituitary secretion of LH, and an increased liver SHBG production seem to be the mechanisms that mediate metformin effect on hyperandrogenism.

On the other hand, other studies compared metformin effects to those obtained from oral contraceptives or anti-androgen drugs: the latter achieved more effective results on hyperandrogenism than metformin alone [201].

4.6   Cosmetic Approaches

Cosmetic methods are widely used and can be categorized as short-term and long-term [225]. Short-term mechanical methods include shaving, chemical depilation, waxing, and bleaching. Long-term mechanical methods include:

- Electrolysis: galvanic electrolysis facilitates chemical destruction of the dermal papilla; thermolytic electrolysis induces heat injury of the hair follicle in the treated area; blended electrolysis includes the synergetic application of both energies [226].
- Laser therapy: it is based on selective photo-thermolysis, wherein melanin of hair follicles accumulates the light energy, which in turn destroys the hair bulb [227]. Four to six treatments are required to achieve a desired effect.
- Intense pulse light therapy: radiofrequency can be used in women with blond hair and light skin, when lasers are not effective [226].

A 13.9% topical solution of eflornithine hydrochloride (HCL) can be used to reduce facial hair growth. It acts as permanent inhibitor of enzyme ornithine decarboxylase, which is required for the growth and differentiation of cells in the hair follicle. This action is reversible and hirsutism relapsed after 8 weeks of cessation of treatment; its use is not approved for large surface areas of the skin due to systemic effects; thus it should be used only for the removal of facial hair [228]. It is not available in every European country. A topical preparation, eflornithine hydrochloride cream 13.9%, is approved in many countries for the treatment of unwanted facial hair in women; it does not remove hair, but acts to reduce the rate of hair growth [229]. Systemic absorption is extremely low; side effects include itching and dry skin [230, 231].

4.7 Treatment Protocols

4.7.1 Acne

In patients with acne who fail to respond to topical therapies, OCs with anti-androgenic properties are recommended as top therapy (level of evidence IA) over oral antibiotic therapy [3].

The improvement in acne is attributed to a significant reduction in sebum production in those areas of the skin that have sebaceous glands [23, 232].

The improvement in skin health suggests that the estrogenic stimulation of the body under EPs may improve the grade of skin hydration [166]. This effect is probably due to an estrogen action on glycosaminoglycans (and acid mucopolysaccharides) and, especially, on hyaluronic acid synthesis in the skin; these molecules are able to increase cutaneous water content under estrogenic stimulation [233–235].

OCPs are effective in the treatment of acne, with studies demonstrating 40–70% reduction in lesion counts [24].

Some authors suggest the addition of spironolactone 50 mg per day (level of evidence IB) after 3 months of insufficient treatment with OC [3].

Spironolactone is not FDA approved for the indication of acne, but spironolactone alone or combined with OCPs is effective in 33–85% reduction in acne lesion counts and also improves seborrhea [53].

Oral antibiotics are often offered as adjunctive treatment, particularly for the cure of pustular acne [3, 236].

The use of flutamide is considered an off-label second-line therapy, usually when some contraindications are present to the use of EP.

When used for the treatment of mild or moderate acne, flutamide should be prescribed at lower doses: a daily dose of 125 mg seems to be effective [15].

In young teenagers with PCOS who were not at risk of pregnancy, combined therapy with a minidose of flutamide and metformin [237] resulted superior to monotherapy with a fourth-generation OCP [238].

A daily dose of finasteride 5 mg is not recommended for the treatment of acne, because it is less effective than flutamide [6, 174].

Long-term targets of care should be established at the beginning of the relationship between PCOS patients and physician, especially for those aspects regarding the family planning, acceptance of systemic and specifically hormonal therapy, and expectations of length of therapy. Frequent evaluation initially is very useful, because it increases patient's compliance to the therapy and enables monitoring and management of undesired adverse effects [53].

4.7.2 Hirsutism

Decrease of ovarian androgen production is commonly obtained by EP administration. OCP therapy is recommended for 2 years, and it has been shown that suppression of serum androgens can continue for up to 2 years after stopping treatment [153]. The use of OCPs containing cyproterone acetate, drospirenone [5], and dienogest is greatly suggested.

A period of 6 months is usually adequate to observe initial benefits in body and limb hair reduction. On the contrary, facial hair may take almost a couple of years of therapy to show improvement [239].

Patients should be educated that response to systemic therapy is slow, in order to improve their compliance to the treatment protocol [63].

After 6 months of therapy with OCPs only, some authors suggest to introduce spironolactone [176, 196, 240] or flutamide or finasteride, if patients do not report any improvement.

Spironolactone should be given for at least 6 months to obtain maximum improvement in hirsutism [5].

Lower doses of flutamide (62.5 mg daily) and finasteride (2.5 mg daily) have shown equal efficacy at improving hirsutism, but with decreased costs and side effects [5].

The efficacy of OCP treatment of hirsutism might be reduced in obese patients (50% of PCOS patients) [241, 242].

An interesting study demonstrated that obese PCOS women did not have any improvement in hirsutism after 6 months of OCP treatment, compared to a clinically significant change in androgen levels and Ferriman-Gallwey score in lean PCOS patients [241].

In this kind of patients the association of EP with an anti-androgenic agent could be more successful, even if there are no clear specific data on obese PCOS women [5].

Cosmetic treatments should be encouraged because they complete the effect of anti-androgen therapy: the only permanent method of hair removal is electrolysis or laser.

4.7.3   Alopecia: Defluvium

There are no extensive trials for alopecia, but OCPs and androgen blockers are usually given in association [242, 243], especially finasteride as first choice and then flutamide as second-line treatment.

The treatment period to achieve a significant result is usually 18–24 months. Besides systemic treatment, alopecia can be controlled with topical minoxidil 2% or 5% and, if necessary, with hair transplant [244, 245].

Acknowledgments   A special thanks goes to my advisor Prof. Lilliana Ciotta (University of Catania), who has been a constant guide in the complex world of gynecological endocrinology.

Conflict of interest: The author declares no potential conflict of interest with respect to research, authorship, and/or publication of this article.

References

1. Vrbikova J, Cibula D. Combined oral contraceptives in the treatment of polycystic ovary syndrome. Hum Reprod Update. 2005;11:277–91.

2. Yildiz BO. Oral contraceptives in polycystic ovary syndrome: risk-benefit assessment. Semin Reprod Med. 2008;26:111–20.
3. Buzney E, Sheu J, Buzney C, Reynolds R. Polycystic ovary syndrome: a review for dermatologist. J Am Acad Dermatol. 2014;71:859.e1–859.e15.
4. Azziz R. The evaluation and management of hirsutism. Obstet Gynecol. 2003;101:995–1007.
5. Archer JS, Chang RJ. Hirsutism and acne in polycystic ovary syndrome. Best Pract Res Clin Obstet Gynaecol. 2004;18(5):737–54.
6. Bowles SM, Mills RJ. Sex hormone binding globulin: effect of synthetic steroids on the assay and effect of oral contraceptives. Ann Clin Biochem. 1981;18:226–31.
7. Stanczyk FZ. All progestins are not created equal. Steroids. 2003;68:879–90.
8. Mes-Krowinkel MG, Louwers YV, Mulders AG, de Jong FH, Fauser BC, Laven JS. Influence of oral contraceptives on anthropomorphometric, endocrine, and metabolic profiles of anovulatory polycystic ovary syndrome patients. Fertil Steril. 2014;101(6):1757–65.
9. De Leo V, Di Sabatino A, Musacchio MC, Morgante G, Scolaro V, Cianci A, Petraglia F. Effect of oral contraceptives on markers of hyperandrogenism and SHBG in women with polycystic ovary syndrome. Contraception. 2010;82:276–80.
10. Alsina JC. After 50 years of ethinylestradiol, another oestrogen in combined oral contraceptives. Eur J Contracept Reprod Health Care. 2010;15:1–3.
11. Lello S, Cavani A. Ethinylestradiol 20 mcg plus Levonorgestrel 100 mcg: clinical pharmacology. Int J Endocrinol. 2014;2014:102184.
12. Batukan C, Muderris II, Ozcelik B, Ozturk A. Comparison of two oral contraceptives containing either drospirenone or cyproterone acetate in the treatment of hirsutism. Gynecol Endocrinol. 2007;23(1):38–44.
13. Van Heusden AM, Fauser BC. Activity of the pituitary-ovarian axis in the pill-free interval during use of low-dose combined oral contraceptives. Contraception. 1999;59:237–43.
14. Wiegratz I, Kutschera E, Lee JH, Moore C, Mellinger U, Winkler UH, Kuhl H. Effect of four different oral contraceptives on various sex hormones and serum-binding globulins. Contraception. 2003;67:25–32.
15. Thiboutot D, Chen WC. Update and future of hormonal therapy in acne. Dermatology. 2003;206:57–67.

16. Rosen MP, Breitkopf DM, Nagamani M. A randomized controlled trial of second- versus third-generation oral contraceptives in the treatment of acne vulgaris. Am J Obstet Gynecol. 2003;188:1158–60.

17. Bhattacharya SM, Jha A. Comparative study of the therapeutic effects of oral contraceptive pills containing desogestrel, cyproterone acetate, and drospirenone in patients with polycystic ovary syndrome. Fertil Steril. 2012;98(4):1053–9.

18. Ruchhoft EA, Elkind-Hirsch KE, Malinak R. Pituitary function is altered during the same cycle in women with polycystic ovary syndrome treated with continuous or cyclic oral contraceptives or a gonadotropin-releasing hormone agonist. Fertil Steril. 1996;66:54–60.

19. Van der Spuy ZM, le Roux PA. Cyproterone acetate for hirsutism. Cochrane Database Syst Rev. 2003;(4):CD001125.

20. Dahlgren E, Landin K, Krotkiewski M, et al. Effects of two antiandrogen treatments on hirsutism and insulin sensitivity in women with polycystic ovary syndrome. Hum Reprod. 1998;13:2706–11.

21. Van Vioten WA, van Haselen CW, van Zuuren EJ, et al. The effect of 2 combined oral contraceptives containing either drospirenone or cyproterone acetate on acne and seborrhea. Cutis. 2002;69:2–15.

22. Haider A, Shaw JC. Treatment of acne vulgaris. JAMA. 2004;292:726–35.

23. Rotaru M, Totoianu IG, Sin AI, et al. Study regarding the microscopic aspects of pilo-sebaceous units after antiandrogen treatment in hirsute women. Romanian J Morphol Embryol. 2015;56(1):63–9.

24. Whiting D, Howsden F. Colour atlas of differential diagnosis of hair loss. Cedar Grove, NJ: Carnfield Publishing; 1996.

25. Kuhl H, Jung-Hoffmann C. Pharmakologie der gestagene. In: Kontrazeption. Stuttgart: Thieme; 1999. p. 28–31.

26. Druckmann R. Profile of the progesterone derivative chlormadinone acetate – pharmocodynamic properties and therapeutic applications. Contraception. 2009;79:272–81.

27. Schneider J, Kneip C, Jahnel U. Comparative effects of chlormadinone acetate and its 3alpha- and 3beta-hydroxy metabolites on progesterone, androgen and glucocorticoid receptors. Pharmacology. 2009;84:74–81.

28. Curran MP, Wagstaff AJ. Ethinylestradiol/chlormadinone acetate. Drugs. 2004;64:751–60.

29. Schindler AE, Campagnoli C, Druckmann R, et al. Classification and pharmacology of progestins. Maturitas. 2003;46(Suppl 1):S7–S16.
30. Raudrant D, Rabe T. Progestogens with antiandrogenic properties. Drugs. 2003;63:463–92.
31. Bouchard P. Chlormadinone acetate (CMA) in oral contraception – a new opportunity. Eur J Contracept Reprod Health Care. 2005;10:7–13.
32. Jung-Hoffmann C, Kuhl H. Divergent effects of two low-dose oral contraceptives on sex hormone-binding globulin and free testosterone. Am J Obstet Gynecol. 1987;156:199–203.
33. Schramm G, Heckes B. Switching hormonal contraceptives to a chlormadinone acetate-containing oral contraceptive. The contraceptive Switch Study. Contraception. 2007;76:84–90.
34. Thorneycroft IH. Evolution of progestins. J Reprod Med. 2002;47:975–80.
35. Mathur R, Levin O, Azziz R. Use of ethinylestradiol/drospirenone combination in patients with the polycystic ovary syndrome. Ther Clin Risk Manag. 2008;4(2):487–92.
36. Batukan C, Muderiss II. Efficacy of a new oral contraceptive containing drospirenone and ethinyl estradiol in the long-term treatment of hirsutism. Fertil Steril. 2006;85:436–40.
37. Azziz R, Gay FL, Potter SR, Bradley E Jr, Boots LR. The effects of prolonged hypertestosteronemia on adrenocortical biosynthesis in oophorectomized women. J Clin Endocrinol Metab. 1991;72:1025–30.
38. Azziz R, Carmina E, Dewailly D, Diamanti-Kandarakis E, Escobar-Morreale HF, Futterweit W, et al. Androgen Excess Society. Positions statement: criteria for defining polycystic ovary syndrome as a predominantly hyperandrogenic syndrome: an Androgen Excess Society guideline. J Clin Endocrinol Metab. 2006;91(11):4237–45.
39. Conard J. Biological coagulation findings in third-generation oral contraceptives. Hum Reprod Update. 1999;5(6):672–80.
40. Oelkers W, Foidart JM, Dombrovicz N, Welter A, Heithecker R. Effects of new oral contraceptive containing an antimineralocorticoid progestogen drospirenone on the renin-aldosterone system, body weight, blood pressure, glucose tolerance and lipid metabolism. J Clin Endocrinol Metab. 1995;80:1816–21.
41. Dickerson V. Quality of life issues. J Reprod Med. 2002;47:985–93.
42. Shulman LP. Safety and efficacy of a new oral contraceptive containing drospirenone. J Reprod Med. 2002;47:981–4.

43. Foidart JM, Wuttke W, Bouw GM, Gerlinger C, Heithecker R. A comparative investigation of contraceptive reliability, cycle control and tolerance of two monophasic oral contraceptives containing either drospirenone or desogestrel. Eur J Contracept Reprod Health Care. 2000;5:124–34.

44. Kriplani A, Periyasamy AJ, Agarwal N, Kulshrestha V, Kumar A, Ammini AC. Effect of oral contraceptive containing ethinyl estradiol combined with drospirenone vs. desogestrel on clinical and biochemical parameters in patients with polycystic ovary syndrome. Contraception. 2010;82:139–46.

45. Mancini F, Cianciosi A, Persico N, Facchinetti F, Busacchi P, Battaglia C. Drospirenone and cardiovascular risk in lean and obese polycystic ovary syndrome patients: a pilot study. Am J Obstet Gynecol. 2010;202:169.e1–8.

46. Martin KA, Chang RJ, Ehrmann DA, Ibanez L, Lobo RA, Rosenfield RL, et al. Evaluation and treatment of hirsutism in premenopausal women: an endocrine society clinical practice guideline. J Clin Endocrinol Metab. 2008;93:1105–20.

47. Fauser BC, Tarlatzis BC, Rebar RW, Legro RS, Balen AH, Lobo R, et al. Consensus on women's health aspects of polycystic ovary syndrome (PCOS): the Amsterdam ESHRE/ASRM-Sponsored 3rd PCOS Consensus Workshop Group. Fertil Steril. 2012;97:28–38.e25.

48. Sitruk-Ware R. Pharmacological profile of progestins. Maturitas. 2008;61:151–7.

49. Sitruk-Ware R, Nath A. The use of newer progestins for contraception. Contraception. 2010;82:410–7.

50. Del Marmol V, Teichmann A, Gertsen K. The role of combined oral contraceptives in the management of acne and seborrhea. Eur J Contracept Reprod Health Care. 2004;9:107–24.

51. Di Carlo C, Gargano V, Sparice S, Tommaselli GA, Bifulco G, Nappi C. Effects of an oral contraceptive containing estradiol valerate and dienogest on circulating androgen levels and acne in young patients with PCOS: an observational preliminary study. Gynecol Endocrinol. 2013;29(12):1048–50.

52. Fruzzetti F, Tremollieres F, Bitzer J. An overview of the development of combined oral contraceptives containing estradiol: focus on estradiol valerate/dienogest. Gynecol Endocrinol. 2012;28:400–8.

53. Kamangar F, Shinkai K. Acne in the adult female patient: a practical approach. Int J Dermatol. 2012;51:1162–74.

54. World Health Organization. Acute myocardial infarction and combined oral contraceptives: results of international multicenter case-control study; WHO collaborative study of cardiovascular disease and steroid hormone contraception. Lancet. 1997;349:1202–9.

55. Curtis KM, Mohllajee AP, Martins SL, et al. Combined oral contraceptive use among women with hypertension: a systematic review. Contraception. 2006;73:179–88.

56. Oelkers WK. Effects of estrogens and progesterons on the renin-aldosterone system and blood pressure. Steroids. 1996;61:166–71.

57. Verhaeghe J. Hormonal contraception in women with the metabolic syndrome: a narrative review. Eur J Contracep Reprod Health Care. 2010;15:305–13.

58. World Health Organization. Medical eligibility criteria for contraceptive use. 3rd ed. 2004. Available at: http://www.who.int/reproductive-health/pubblications/mec/index.htm.

59. Battaglia C, Mancini F, Cianciosi A, et al. Vascular risk in young women with polycystic ovary and polycystic ovary syndrome. Obstet Gynecol. 2008;111:385–95.

60. Kebapcilar L, Bilgir O, Taner CE, Kebapcilar AG, Kozaci DL, Alacacioglu A, et al. Oral contraceptives alone and with spironolactone increase sCD40 ligand in PCOS patients. Arch Gynecol Obstet. 2010;281:539–43.

61. Mach F, Schonbeck U, Libby P. CD40 signaling in vascular cells: a key role in atherosclerosis? Atherosclerosis. 1998;137(Suppl):S89–95.

62. Andrè P, Nannizzi-Alaimo L, Prasad SK, Phillips DR. Platelet-derived CD40L: the switch-hitting player of cardiovascular disease. Circulation. 2002;106:896–9.

63. Baldauff NH, Arslanian S. Optimal management of polycystic ovary syndrome in adolescence. Arch Dis Child. 2015;100:1076–83.

64. Yarali H, Yildirir A, Aybar F, et al. Diastolic dysfunction and increased serum homocysteine concentrations may contribute to increased cardiovascular risk in patients with polycystic ovary syndrome. Fertil Steril. 2001;76:511–6.

65. Harmanci A, Cinar N, Bayraktar M, Yildiz BO. Oral contraceptive plus antiandrogen therapy and cardiometabolic risk in polycystic ovary syndrome. Clin Endocrinol (Oxf). 2013;78:120–5.

66. Bingol B, Gunenc Z, Yilmaz M, et al. Effects of hormone replacement therapy on glucose and lipid profiles and on car-

diovascular risk parameters in postmenopausal women. Arch Gynecol Obstet. 2010;281:857–64.

67. Steegers-Theunissen RP, Boers GH, Steegers EA, et al. Effects of sub-50 oral contraceptives on homocysteine metabolism: a preliminary study. Contraception. 1992;45:129–39.

68. Mammen EF. Oral contraceptive pills and hormonal replacement therapy and thromboembolic disease. Hematol Oncol Clin North Am. 2000;14:1045–59.

69. Rosendaal FR. Venous thrombosis: the role of genes, environment and behavior. Hematology Am Soc Hematol Educ Program. 2005:1–12.

70. Soares GM, Vieira CS, de Paula Martins W, dos Reis RM, de Sà FS, Ferriani RA. Metabolic and cardiovascular impact of oral contraceptives in polycystic ovary syndrome. Int J Clin Pract. 2009;63(1):160–9.

71. Van Hylckama Vlieg A, Helmerhorst FM, Vandenbroucke JP, Doggen CJ, Rosendaal FR. The venous thrombotic risk of oral contraceptives, effects of oestrogen dose and progestogen type: results of the MEGA case-control study. BMJ. 2009;339:b2921.

72. Gomes MP, Deitcher SR. Risk of venous thromboembolic disease associated with hormonal contraceptives and hormone replacement therapy: a clinical review. Arch Intern Med. 2004;164:1965–76.

73. Bhattacharya SM, Jha A, DasMukhopadhyay L. Comparison of two contraceptive pills containing drospirenone and 20 μg or 30 μg ethinyl estradiol for polycystic ovary syndrome. Int J Gynecol Obstet. 2016;132:210–3.

74. Lidegaard O, Nielsen LH, Skovlund CW, Skjeldestad FE, Lokkegaard E. Risk of venous thromboembolism from use of oral contraceptives containing different progestogens and oestrogen doses: Danish cohort study, 2001–9. BMJ. 2011;343:d6423.

75. Carmina E. Oral contraceptives and cardiovascular risk in women with polycystic ovary syndrome. J Endocrinol Investig. 2013;36:358–63.

76. Bird ST, Hartzema AG, Brophy JM, Etminan M, Delaney JA. Risk of venous thromboembolism in women with polycystic ovary syndrome: a population-based matched cohort analysis. CMAJ. 2013;185:E115–20.

77. Prieto D, Contreras C, Sanchez A. Endothelial dysfunction, obesity and insulin resistance. Curr Vasc Pharmacol. 2014;12:412–26.

78. Blankenberg S, Barbaux S, Tiret L. Adhesion molecules and atherosclerosis. Atherosclerosis. 2003;170:191–203.

79. Nasiek M, Kos-Kudla B, Ostrowska Z. Plasma concentration of soluble intercellular adhesion molecule-1 in women with polycystic ovary syndrome. Gynecol Endocrinol. 2004;19: 208–15.

80. Vrbikova J, Vankova M, Sramkova D, et al. Intercellular cell adhesion molecule-1 in PCOS; relation to insulin resistance or obesity. Endocr Abstr. 2005;9:76.

81. Diamanti-Kandarakis E, Alexandraki K, Piperi C. Inflammatory and endothelial markers in women with polycystic ovary syndrome. Eur J Clin Investig. 2006;36:691–7.

82. Gonzalez F, Rote NS, Minium J. Evidence of proatherogenic inflammation in polycystic ovary syndrome. Metabolism. 2009;58:954–62.

83. Hu W, Quiao J, Yang Y, et al. Elevated C-reactive protein and monocyte chemoattractant protein-1 in patients with polycystic ovary syndrome. Eur J Obstet Gynecol Reprod Biol. 2011;157:53–6.

84. Atabekoglu CS, Sonmezer M, Ozmen B, et al. Increased monocyte chemoattractant protein-1 levels indicating early vascular damage in lean young PCOS patients. Fertil Steril. 2011;95:295–7.

85. Hu WH, Qiao J, Li MZ. Association of monocyte chemoattractant protein-1 and the clinical characteristics of polycystic ovary syndrome: analysis of 65 cases. Zhonghua Yi Xue Za Zhi. 2007;87:721–4.

86. Hu WH, Qiao J, Zhao SY, et al. Monocyte chemoattractant protein-1 and its correlation with lipoprotein in polycystic ovary syndrome. Beijing Da Xue Xue Bao. 2006;38:487–91.

87. Hayflick JS, Kilgannon P, Gallatin WM. The intercellular adhesion molecule (ICAM) family of proteins. New members and novel functions. Immunol Res. 1998;17:313–27.

88. Yousuf SD, Rashid F, Mattoo T, Shekhar C, Mudassar S, Zargar MA, Ganie MA. Does oral contraceptive pill increase plasma Intercellular Adhesion Molecule-1, Monocyte Chemoattractant Protein-1 and Tumor Necrosis Factor-a levels in women with Polycystic Ovary Syndrome (PCOS): a pilot study. J Pediatr Adolesc Gynecol. 2017;30(1):58–62.

89. Morin-Papunen L, Rautio K, Ruokonen A, et al. Metformin reduces serum C-reactive protein levels in women with polycystic ovary syndrome. J Clin Endocrinol Metab. 2003;88:4649–54.

90. Doring A, Frohlich M, Lowel H, et al. Third generation oral contraceptive use and cardiovascular risk factors. Atherosclerosis. 2004;172:281–6.

91. Tatsumi H, Kitawaki J, Tanaka K, et al. Lack of stimulatory effect of dienogest on the expression of intercellular adhesion molecule-1 and vascular cell adhesion molecule-1 by endothelial cell as compared with other synthetic progestins. Maturitas. 2002;42:287–94.

92. Hemelaar M, van der Mooren MJ, van Baal WM, et al. Effects of transdermal and oral postmenopausal hormone therapy on vascular function: a randomized, placebo-controlled study in healthy postmenopausal women. Menopause. 2005;12:526–35.

93. Seeger H, Petersen G, Schulte-Wintrop E, et al. Effect of two oral contraceptives containing ethinylestradiol and levonorgestrel on serum and urinary surrogate markers of endothelial function. Int J Clin Pharmacol Ther. 2002;40:150–7.

94. Kernohan AF, Spiers A, Sattar N. Effects of low-dose continuous combined HRT on vascular function in women with type 2 diabetes. Diab Vasc Dis Res. 2004;1:82–8.

95. Gomes Valeria A, Vieira CS, Jacob-Ferreira AL, Belo VA, Soares GM, França JB, et al. Oral contraceptive containing chlormadinone acetate and ethinylestradiol reduces plasma concentrations of Matrix Metalloproteinase-2 in women with polycystic ovary syndrome. Basic Clin Pharmacol Toxicol. 2012;111:211–6.

96. Gomes VA, Vieira CS, Jacob-Ferreira AL, Belo VA, Soares GM, Fernandes JB, et al. Imbalanced circulating matrix metalloproteinases in polycystic ovary syndrome. Mol Cell Biochem. 2011;353:251–7.

97. Ridker PM, Hennekens CH, Buring JE, et al. C-reactive protein and other markers of inflammation in the prediction of cardiovascular disease in women. N Engl J Med. 2000;342:836–43.

98. Orio F Jr, Palomba S, Di Biase S, et al. Homocysteine levels and C677T polymorphism of methylenetetrahydrofolate reductase in women with polycystic ovary syndrome. J Clin Endocrinol Metab. 2003;88:673–9.

99. Toulis KA, Goulis DG, Mintziori G, et al. Meta-analysis of cardiovascular disease risk markers in women with polycystic ovary syndrome. Hum Reprod Update. 2011;17:741–60.

100. Van Rooijen M, Hansson LO, Frostegard J, et al. Treatment with combined oral contraceptives induces a rise in serum C-reactive protein in the absence of a general inflammatory response. J Thromb Haemost. 2006;4:77–82.

101. Chen MJ, Yang WA, Chen HF, et al. Increased follistatin levels after oral contraceptives treatment in obese and non-

obese women with polycystic ovary syndrome. Hum Reprod. 2010;25:779–85.

102. Teede HJ, Meyer C, Hutchison SK, et al. Endothelial function and insulin resistance in polycystic ovary syndrome: the effects of medical therapy. Fertil Steril. 2010;93:184–91.

103. Cauci S, Di Santolo M, Culhane JF, et al. Effects of third-generation oral contraceptives on high-sensitivity C-reactive protein and homocysteine in young women. Obstet Gynecol. 2008;111:857–64.

104. Yildizhan R, Gokce AI, Yildizhan B, Cim N. Comparison of the effects of chlormadinone acetate versus drospirenone containing oral contraceptives on metabolic and hormonal parameters in women with PCOS for a period of two-year follow-up. Gynecol Endocrinol. 2015;31(5):396–400.

105. Chang K, Weiss D, Suo J, Vega JD, Giddens D, Taylor WR, Jo H. Bone morphogenic protein antagonists are coexpressed with bone morphogenic protein 4 in endothelial cells exposed to unstable flow in vitro in mouse aortas and in human coronary arteries: role of bone morphogenic protein antagonists in inflammation and atherosclerosis. Circulation. 2007;116:1258–66.

106. Dohi T, Ejima C, Kato R, Kawamura YI, Kawashima R, Mizutani N, et al. Therapeutic potential of follistatin for colonic inflammation in mice. Gastroenterology. 2005;128:411–23.

107. Orio F, Palomba S, Cascella T, Simone BD, Biade SD, Russo T, et al. Early impairment of endothelial structure and function in young normal-weight women with polycystic ovary syndrome. J Clin Endocrinol Metab. 2004;89:4588–93.

108. Gode F, Karagoz C, Posaci C, Saatli B, Uysal D, Secil M, Akdeniz B. Alteration of cardiovascular risk parameters in women with polycystic ovary syndrome who were prescribed to ethinylestradiol-cyproterone acetate. Arch Gynecol Obstet. 2011;284:923–9.

109. Korytkowski MT, Mokan M, Horwitz MJ, Berga S. Metabolic effects of oral contraceptives in women with polycystic ovary syndrome. J Clin Endocrinol Metab. 1995;80:3327–34.

110. Luque-Ramirez M, Medieta-Azcona C, del Rey Sanchez JM, Maties M. Effects of an antiandrogenic oral contraceptive pill compared with metformin on blood coagulation tests and endothelial function in women with the polycystic ovary syndrome: influence of obesity and smoking. Eur J Endocrinol. 2009;160:469–80.

111. Cogliano V, Grosse Y, Baan R, Straif K, Secretan B, ElGhissassi F, WHO International Agency for Research on Cancer. Carcinogenicity of combined oestrogen-progestagen contraceptives and menopausal treatment. Lancet Oncol. 2005;6:552–3.

112. Gottschau M, Kjaer SK, Jensen A, Munk C, Mellemkjaer L. Risk of cancer among women with polycystic ovary syndrome: a Danish Cohort study. Gynecol Oncol. 2015;136:99–103.

113. Cowan L, Gordis L, Tonascia JA, Jones GS. Breast cancer incidence in women with a history of progesterone deficiency. Am J Epidemiol. 1981;114:209–17.

114. Giammon MD, Thompson WD. Polycystic ovaries and the risk of breast cancer. Am J Epidemiol. 1991;134:818–24.

115. Barry JA, Azizia MM, Hardiman PJ. Risk of endometrial, ovarian and breast cancer in women with polycystic ovary syndrome: a systematic review and meta-analysis. Hum Reprod Update. 2014;20:748–58.

116. Chittenden BG, Fullerton G, Maheshwari A, Bhattacharya S. Polycystic ovary syndrome and the risk of gynecological cancer: a systematic review. Reprod Biomed Online. 2009;19:398–405.

117. Pike MC, Spicer DV. Hormonal contraception and chemoprevention of female cancers. Endocr Relat Cancer. 2000;7(2):73–83.

118. Jordan S, Wilson L, Nagle CM, Green AC, Olsen CM, Bain CJ, et al. Cancers in Australia in 2010 attributable to and prevented by the use of combined oral contraceptives. Aust N Z J Public Health. 2015;39:441–5.

119. Halperin IJ, Kumar SS, Stroup DF, Laredo SE. The association between the combined oral contraceptive pill and insulin resistance, dysglycemia and dyslipidemia in women with polycystic ovary syndrome: a systematic review and meta-analysis of observational studies. Hum Reprod. 2011;26:191–201.

120. Apridonidze T, Essah PA, Iuorno MJ, Nestler JE. Prevalence and characteristics of the metabolic syndrome in women with polycystic ovary syndrome. J Clin Endocrinol Metab. 2005;90:1929–35.

121. Maier P, Spritzer PM. Aromatase gene polymorphism does not influence clinical phenotype and response to oral contraceptive pills in polycystic ovary syndrome women. Gynecol Obstet Investig. 2012;74:136–42.

122. Cerel-Suhl SL, Yeager BF. Update on oral contraceptive pills. Am Fam Physician. 1999;60:2073–84.

123. Morin-Papunen LC, Vauhkonen I, Koivunen RM, Ruokonen A, Tapanainen JS. Insulin sensitivity, insulin secretion, and metabolic and hormonal parameters in healthy women and women with polycystic ovarian syndrome. Hum Reprod. 2000;15:1266–74.

124. Crook D, Godsland I. Safety evaluation of modern oral contraceptives. Contraception. 1998;57:189–201.

125. Lopez LM, Grimes DA, Schulz KF. Steroidal contraceptives: effect on carbohydrate metabolism in women without diabetes mellitus. Cochrane Database Syst Rev. 2009;(4):CD006133.

126. Godsland IF, Crook D, Simpson R, Proudler T, Felton C, Lees B, et al. The effects of different formulations of oral contraceptive agents on lipid and carbohydrate metabolism. N Engl J Med. 1990;323:1375–81.

127. Diamanti-Kandarakis E, Baillargeon JP, Iuorno MJ, Jakubowicz DJ, Nestler JE. A modern medical quandary: polycystic ovary syndrome, insulin resistance and oral contraceptive pill. J Clin Endocrinol Metab. 2003;88:1927–32.

128. Nader S, Diamanti-Kandarakis E. Polycystic ovary syndrome, oral contraceptives and metabolic issues: new perspectives and a unifying hypothesis. Hum Reprod. 2007;22:317–22.

129. Adeniji AA, Essah PA, Nestler J, Cheang KI. Metabolic effects of a commonly used combined hormonal oral contraceptive in women with and without polycystic ovary syndrome. J Womens Health (Larchmt). 2016;25:638–45.

130. Battaglia C, Mancini F, Fabbri R, Persico N, Busacchi P, Facchinetti F, Venturoli S. Polycystic ovary syndrome and cardiovascular risk in young patients treated with drospirenone-ethinylestradiol or contraceptive vaginal ring. A prospective, randomized, pilot study. Fertil Steril. 2010;94:1417–25.

131. Romualdi D, De Cicco S, Busacca M, Gagliano D, Lanzone A, Guido M. Clinical efficacy and metabolic impact of two different dosages of ethinyl-estradiol in association with drospirenone in normal-weight women with polycystic ovary syndrome: a randomized study. J Endocrinol Investig. 2013;36(8):636–41.

132. Guido M, Romualdi D, Giuliani M, et al. Drospirenone for the treatment of hirsute women with polycystic ovary syndrome: a clinical, endocrinological, metabolic pilot study. J Clin Endocrinol Metab. 2004;89:2817–23.

133. Kraus D, Jager J, Meier B, et al. Aldosterone inhibits uncoupling protein-1, induces insulin resistance, and stimulates pro-inflammatory adipokines in adipocytes. Horm Metab Res. 2005;37:455–9.

134. Corry DB, Tuck ML. The effect of aldosterone on glucose metabolism. Curr Hypertens Rep. 2003;5:106–9.

135. Fruzzetti F, Perini D, Lazzarini V, et al. Comparison of effects of 3 mg drospirenone plus 20 μg ethinyl estradiol alone or combined with metformin or cyproterone acetate on classic metabolic cardiovascular risk factors in nonobese women with polycystic ovary syndrome. Fertil Steril. 2010;94:1793–8.

136. Cullberg G, Hamberger L, Mattsson LA, Mobacken H, Samsioe G. Lipid metabolic studies in women with a polycystic ovary syndrome during treatment with a low-dose desogestrel-ethinylestradiol combination. Acta Obstet Gynecol Scand. 1985;64:203–7.

137. Rojanasakul A, Chailurkit L, Sirimongkolkasem R, Chaturachinda K. Effects of combined desogestrel-ethinylestradiol treatment on lipid profiles in women with polycystic ovarian syndrome. Fertil Steril. 1987;48:581–5.

138. Escobar-Morreale HF, Lasuncion MA, Sancho J. Treatment of hirsutism with ethinylestradiol-desogestrel contraceptive pills has beneficial effects on the lipid profile and improves insulin sensitivity. Fertil Steril. 2000;74:816–9.

139. NIH Consensus Conference. Triglyceride, high-density lipoprotein and coronary heart disease. NIH Consensus Development Panel on triglyceride, high-density lipoprotein, and coronary heart disease. JAMA. 1993;269(4):505–10.

140. Sagsoz N, Orbak Z, Noyan V, Yucel A, Ucar B, Yildiz L. The effects of oral contraceptives including low-dose estrogen and drospirenone on the concentration of leptin and ghrelin in polycystic ovary syndrome. Fertil Steril. 2009;92:660–6.

141. Prelevic GM, Wurzburger MI, Trpkovic D. Effects of a low dose estrogen-antiandrogen combination (Diane-35) on lipid and carbohydrate metabolism in patients with polycystic ovary syndrome. Gynecol Endocrinol. 1990;4:157–68.

142. Wild RA. Metabolic aspects of polycystic ovary syndrome. Semin Reprod Endocrinol. 1997;15:105–10.

143. Talbott E, Guzick D, Clerici A, Berga S, Detre K, Wiemer K, Kuller L. Coronary heart disease risk factors in women with polycystic ovary syndrome. Arterioscler Thromb Vasc Biol. 1995;15:821–6.

144. Wild RA, Painter PC, Coulson PB, Carruth KB, Ranney GB. Lipoprotein lipid concentrations and cardiovascular risk in women with polycystic ovary syndrome. J Clin Endocrinol Metab. 1985;61:946–51.

145. Ehrmann DA. Polycystic ovary syndrome. N Engl J Med. 2005;352:1223–36.

146. Michael H, Harkonen PL, Vaananen HK, Hentunen TA. Estrogen and testosterone use different cellular pathways to inhibit osteoclastogenesis and bone resorption. J Bone Miner Res. 2005;20:2224–32.

147. Vessey M, Mant J, Painter R. Oral contraception and other factors in relation to hospital referral for fracture. Findings in a large cohort study. Contraception. 1998;57:231–5.

148. Moran LJ, Thomson RL, Buckley JD, Noakes M, Clifton PM, Norman RJ, Brinkworth GD. Steroidal contraceptive use is associated with lower bone mineral density in polycystic ovary syndrome. Endocrine. 2015;50:811–5.

149. Kassanos D, Trakakis E, Baltas CS, Papakonstantinou O, Simeonidis G, Salamalekis G, et al. Augmentation of cortical bone mineral density in women with polycystic ovary syndrome: a peripheral quantitative computed tomography (pQCT) study. Hum Reprod. 2010;25:2107–14.

150. Yang J, Zhang X, Wang W, Liu J. Insulin stimulates osteoblast proliferation and differentiation through ERK and PI3K in MG-63 cells. Cell Biochem Funct. 2010;28:334–41.

151. Speroff L, Glass RH, Kase NG. Hirsutism. In: Speroff L, Glass RH, Kase NG, editors. Clinical gynecologic endocrinology and infertility. 6th ed. Baltimore: Williams and Wilkins; 1999. p. 523–56.

152. Farquhar C, Lee O, Toomath R, Jepson R. Spironolactone versus placebo or in combination with steroids for hirsutism and/or acne (Cochrane Review). The Cochrane Library Issue 4. Chichester: Wiley; 2003.

153. Lobo RA, Shoupe D, Serafini P, Brinton D, Horton R. The effects of two doses of spironolactone on serum androgens and anagen hair in hirsute women. Fertil Steril. 1985;43:200–5.

154. Muhn P, Krattenmacher R, Beier S, Elger W, Schillinger E. Drospirenone: a novel progestogen with antimineralocorticoid and antiandrogenic activity. Pharmacological characterization in animal models. Contraception. 1995;51:99–110.

155. Shaw JC, White LE. Long-term safety of spironolactone in acne: results of an 8-year follow up study. J Cutan Med Surg. 2002;6:541–5.
156. Mackenzie IS, Macdonald TM, Thompson A, Morant S, Wei L. Spironolactone and risk of incident breast cancer in women older than 55 years: retrospective, marched cohort study. BMJ. 2012;345:e4447.
157. Karakurt F, Sahin I, Guler S, Demirbas B, Culha C, Serter R, Aral Y. Comparison of the clinical efficacy of flutamide and spironolactone plus ethinylestradiol/cyproterone acetate in the treatment of hirsutism: a randomized controlled study. Adv Ther. 2008;25(4):321–8.
158. Diamanti-Kandarakis E, Economou FN, Livadas E, Tantalaki E, Piperi C, Papavassiliou AG, Panidis D. Hyperreninemia characterizing women with polycystic ovary syndrome improves after metformin therapy. Kidney Blood Press Res. 2009;32:24–31.
159. Studen KB, Sebestjen M, Pfeifer M, Prezelj J. Influence of spironolactone treatment on endothelial function in non-obese women with polycystic ovary syndrome. Eur J Endocrinol. 2011;164:389–95.
160. Diamanti-Kandarakis E, Alexandraki K, Protogerou A, Piperi C, Papamichael C, Aessopos A, et al. Metformin administration improves endothelial function in women with polycystic ovary syndrome. Eur J Endocrinol. 2005;152:749–56.
161. Cascella T, Palomba S, Tauchmanova L, Manguso F, DiBiase S, Labella D, et al. Serum aldosterone concentration and cardiovascular risk in women with polycystic ovary syndrome. J Clin Endocrinol Metab. 2006;91:4395–400.
162. Romualdi D, Costantini B, Selvaggi L, Giuliani M, Cristello F, Macri F, et al. Metformin improves endothelial function in normoinsulinemic PCOS patients: a new perspective. Hum Reprod. 2008;23:2127–33.
163. Fujimoto R, Morimoto I, Morita E, Sugimoto H, Yto Y, Eto S. Androgen receptors, 5α-reductase activity and androgen-dependent proliferation of vascular smooth muscle cells. J Steroid Biochem Mol Biol. 1994;50:169–74.
164. Hutchison SJ, Sudhir K, Chou TM, Sievers RE, Zhu BQ, Sun YP, et al. Testosterone worsens endothelial dysfunction associated with hypercholesterolemia and environmental tobacco smoke exposure in male rabbit aorta. J Am Coll Cardiol. 1997;29:800–7.

165. Lee AT, Zane LT. Dermatologic manifestations of polycystic ovary syndrome. Am J Clin Dermatol. 2007;8:201–19.

166. Colonna L, Pacifico V, Lello S, Sorge R, Raskovic D, Primavera G. Skin improvement with two different oestroprogestins in patients affected by acne and polycystic ovary syndrome: clinical and instrumental evaluation. J Eur Acad Dermatol Venereol. 2012;26:1364–71.

167. Wong IL, Morris RS, Chang L, et al. A prospective randomized trial comparing finasteride to spironolactone in the treatment of hirsute women. J Clin Endocrinol Metab. 1995;80:233–8.

168. Bayram F, Muderris BF II, Guven M, Kelestimur F. Comparison of high dose finasteride (5 mg-day) versus low-dose finasteride (2.5 mg/day) in the treatment of hirsutism. Eur J Endocrinol. 2002;147:467–71.

169. Muderris BF II, Guven M, Kelestimur F. Comparison of high dose finasteride (5 mg/day) versus low-dose finasteride (2.5 mg/day) in the treatment of hirsutism. Eur J Endocrinol. 2002;147:467–71.

170. Falsetti L, Gambera A, Legrenzi L, Iacobello C, Bugari G. Comparison of finasteride versus flutamide in the treatment of hirsutism. Eur J Endocrinol. 1999;141:361–7.

171. Tartagni M, Schonauer LM, De Salvia MA, et al. Comparison of Diane 35 and Diane 35 plus finasteride in the treatment of hirsutism. Fertil Steril. 2000;73:718.

172. Castello R, Tosi F, Perrone F, et al. Outcome of long term treatment with the 5α-reductase inhibitor finasteride in idiopathic hirsutism: clinical and hormonal effects during a 1 year course of therapy and 1 year follow-up. Fertil Steril. 1996;66:734.

173. Tartagni MV, Alrasheed H, Damiani GR, Montagnani M, De Salvia M, De Pergola G, et al. Intermittent low-dose finasteride administration is effective for treatment of hirsutism in adolescent girls: a pilot study. J Pediatr Adolesc Gynecol. 2014;27:161–5.

174. Carmina E, Lobo RA. A comparison of the relative efficacy of antiandrogens for the treatment of acne in hyperandrogenic women. Clin Endocrinol. 2002;57:231–4.

175. Muderris B II, Ayram F. Clinical efficacy of lower dose flutamide 125 mg/day in the treatment of hirsutism. J Endocrinol Investig. 1999;22:165–8.

176. Moghetti P, Tosi F, Tosti A, et al. Comparison of spironolactone, flutamide, and finasteride efficacy in the treatment of hirsut-

ism: a randomized, double blind, placebo-controlled trial. J Clin Endocrinol. 2000;85:89–94.

177. Vrbikova J, Hill M, Dvorakova K, Stanicka S, Vondra K, Starka L. Flutamide suppresses adrenal steroidogenesis but has no effect on insulin resistance and secretion and lipid levels in overweight women with polycystic ovary syndrome. Gynecol Obstet Investig. 2004;58:36–41.

178. Couzinet B, Pholsena M, Young J, Schaison G. The impact of a pure anti-androgen (flutamide) on LH, FSH, androgens and clinical status in idiopathic hirsutism. Clin Endocrinol. 1993;39:157–62.

179. Paradisi R, Fabbri R, Battaglia C, Venturoli S. Ovulatory effects of flutamide in the polycystic ovary syndrome. Gynecol Endocrinol. 2013;29(4):391–5.

180. Paradisi R, Venturoli S. Retrospective observational study on the effects and tolerability of flutamide in a large population of patients with various kinds of hirsutism over a 15-year period. Eur J Endocrinol. 2010;163:139–47.

181. Eagleson CA, Gingrich MB, Pastor CL, et al. Polycystic ovarian syndrome: evidence that flutamide restores sensitivity of the gonadotropin-releasing hormone pulse generator to inhibition by estradiol and progesterone. J Clin Endocrinol Metab. 2000;85:4047–52.

182. Brodgen RN, Clissold SP. Flutamide: a preliminary review of its pharmacodynamics and pharmacokinetic properties and therapeutic efficacy in advanced prostatic cancer. Drugs. 1989;38:185–203.

183. Muderris II, Bayram F, Guven M. Treatment of hirsutism with lowest-dose flutamide (62.5 mg/day). Gynecol Endocrinol. 2000;14:38–41.

184. Diamanti-Kandarakis E, Mitrakou A, Hennes MM, Platanissiotis D, Kaklas N, Spina J, et al. Insulin sensitivity and antiandrogenic therapy in women with polycystic ovary syndrome. Metabolism. 1995;44:525–31.

185. De Leo V, la Marca A, Lanzetta D, Cariello PL, D'Antona D, Morgante G. Effects of flutamide on pituitary and adrenal responsiveness to corticotrophin releasing factor. Clin Endocrinol. 1998;49:85–9.

186. Ibanez L, Potau N, Marcos MV, de Zegher F. Treatment of hirsutism, hyperandrogenism, oligomenorrhea, dyslipidemia and hyperinsulinism in nonobese, adolescent girls: effect of flutamide. J Clin Endocrinol Metab. 2000;85:3251–5.

187. Moghetti P, Tosi F, Castello R, Magnani CM, Negri C, Brun E, et al. The insulin resistance in women with hyperandrogenism is partially reversed by antiandrogen treatment: evidence that androgens impair insulin action in women. J Clin Endocrinol Metab. 1996;81:952–60.

188. Dodin S, Faurc N, Cedrin I, Mcchain C, Turcot-Lemay L, Guy J, Lemay A. Clinical efficacy and safety of low-dose flutamide alone and combined with an oral contraceptive for the treatment of idiopathic hirsutism. Clin Endocrinol. 1995;43:575–82.

189. Diamanti-Kandarakis E, Mitrakou A, Raptis S, Tolis G, Duleba AJ. The effect of a pure antiandrogen receptor blocker, flutamide, on the lipid profile in the polycystic ovary syndrome. J Clin Endocrinol Metab. 1998;83:2699–705.

190. Sahin I, Serter R, Karakurt F, Demirbas B, Guler S, Culha C, et al. Leptin levels increase during flutamide therapy in women with polycystic ovary syndrome. Horm Res. 2003;60:232–6.

191. Gomez JL, Dupont A, Cusan L, Tremblay M, et al. Incidence of liver toxicity associated with the use of flutamide in prostate cancer patients. Am J Med. 1992;92:465–70.

192. Ibanez L, Jaramillo A, Ferrer A, Zegher F. Absence of hepatotoxicity after long term, low dose flutamide in hyperandrogenic girls and young women. Hum Reprod. 2005;20(7):1833–6.

193. Dikensoy E, Balat O, Pence S, Akcali C, Cicek H. The risk of hepatotoxicity during long-term and low-dose flutamide treatment in hirsutism. Arch Gynecol Obstet. 2009;279:321–7.

194. Takashima E, Iguchu K, Usut S, Yamamoto H, et al. Metabolite profiles in serum from patients with flutamide-induced hepatic dysfunction. Biol Pharm Bull. 2003;26:1455–60.

195. Muderris II, Bayram F, Guven M. A prospective, randomized trial comparing flutamide (250 mg/d) and finasteride (5 mg/d) in the treatment of hirsutism. Fertil Steril. 2000;73:984–7.

196. Cusan L, Dupont A, Gomez JL, Tremblay RR, Labrie F. Comparison of flutamide and spironolactone in the treatment of hirsutism: a randomized controlled trial. Fertil Steril. 1994;61:281–7.

197. Azziz R, Dewailly D. Diagnosis, screening and treatment of nonclassic 21-hydroxylase deficiency. Lippincott: Raven Press; 1997. p. 181–92.

198. Catteau-Jonard S, Cortet Rudelli C, et al. Hyperandrogenism in adolescent girls. Endocrin Dev. 2012;22:181–93.

199. Parker LN. Control of adrenal androgen secretion. Endocrinol Metab Clin North Am. 1991;20:401–21.
200. Carmina E, Dewailly D, Escobar-Morreale H, et al. Non-classic congenital adrenal hyperplasia due to 21-hydroxylase deficiency revisited: an update with a special focus on adolescent and adult women. Hum Reprod Update. 2017;23(5):580–99.
201. Stracquadanio M, Ciotta L. Metabolic aspects of PCOS. 2015. ISBN: 978-3-319-16759-6.
202. Jenkins D, Wolever T, Bacon S. Diabetic diets: high carbohydrate combined with high fiber. Am J Clin Nutr. 1980;33(8):1729–33.
203. Simpson HC, Simpson RW, Lousley S, et al. A high carbohydrate leguminous fiber diet improves all aspects of diabetic control. Lancet. 1981;1(8210):1–5.
204. Wild RA, Carmina E, Diamanti-Kandarakis E, et al. Assessment of cardiovascular risk and prevention of cardiovascular disease in women with the polycystic ovary syndrome: a consensus statement by the Androgen Excess and Polycystic Ovary Syndrome (AE-PCOS) Society. J Clin Endocrinol Metab. 2010;95:2038–49.
205. Aubuchon M, Kunselman AR, Schlaff WD, et al. Metformin and/or clomiphene do not adversely affect liver or renal function in women with polycystic ovary syndrome. J Clin Endocrinol Metab. 2011;96(10):E1645–9.
206. Attia GR, Rainey WE, Carr BR. Metformin directly inhibits androgen production in human thecal cells. Fertil Steril. 2001;76:517–24.
207. Preiss D, Sattar N, Harborne L, et al. The effects of 8 months of metformin on circulating GGT and ALT levels in obese women with polycystic ovarian syndrome. Int J Clin Pract. 2008;62:1337–43.
208. Palomba S, Falbo A, Russo T, et al. Insulin sensitivity after metformin suspension in normal-weight women with polycystic ovary syndrome. J Clin Endocrinol Metab. 2007;92:3128–35.
209. Aruna J, Mittal S, Kumar S, et al. Metformin therapy in women with polycystic ovary syndrome. Int J Gynaecol Obstet. 2004;87:237–41.
210. Glueck CJ, Wang P, Fontaine R, et al. Metformin to restore normal menses in oligo-amenorrheic teenage girls with polycystic ovary syndrome (PCOS). J Adolesc Health. 2001;29:160–9.
211. Azziz R, Ehrmann D, Legro RS, et al. Troglitazone improves ovulation and hirsutism in the polycystic ovary syndrome:

a multicenter, double blind, placebo-controlled trial. J Clin Endocrinol Metab. 2001;86:1626–32.

212. ASRM Practice Committee. Insulin-sensitizing agents in PCOS. Fertil Steril. 2008:S69–S73.

213. Antonucci T, Whitcomb R, McLain R, et al. Impaired glucose tolerance is normalized by treatment with the thiazolidinedione troglitazone. Diabetes Care. 1998;20:188–93.

214. Palomba S, Falbo A, Zullo F, Orio F. Evidence-based and potential benefits of metformin in the polycystic ovary syndrome: a comprehensive review. Endocr Rev. 2009;30(1):1–50.

215. Farshchi H, Taylor M, Macdonald I. Deleterious effects of omitting breakfast on insulin sensitivity and fasting lipid profiles in healthy lean women. Am J Clin Nutr. 2005;81:388–96.

216. Dunn CJ, Peters DH. Metformin. A review of its pharmacological properties and therapeutic use in non-insulin-dependent diabetes mellitus. Drugs. 1995;49:721–49.

217. Palomba S, Falbo A, Orio F, et al. Efficacy predictors for metformin and clomiphene citrate treatment in anovulatory infertile patients with polycystic ovary syndrome. Fertil Steril. 2008;91:2557–67. https://doi.org/10.1016/j.fertnstert.2008.03.011.

218. Maciel GAR, Soares Junior JM, Leme Alves da Motta E, et al. Nonobese women with polycystic ovary syndrome respond better than obese women to treatment with metformin. Fertil Steril. 2004;81(2):355–60.

219. Mathur R, Alexander CJ, Yano J, et al. Use of metformin in polycystic ovary syndrome. Am J Obstet Gynecol. 2008;199(6):596–609.

220. Liu S, Willett WC, Stampfer MJ, et al. A prospective study of dietary glycemic load, carbohydrate intake and risk of coronary heart disease in US women. Am J Clin Nutr. 2000;71:1455–61.

221. Legro RS, Barnhart HX, Schlaff WD, et al. Clomiphene, metformin, or both for infertility in the polycystic ovary syndrome. N Engl J Med. 2007;356:551–66.

222. Deplewski D, Rosenfield RL. Role of hormones in pilosebaceous unit development. Endocr Rev. 2000;21:363–92.

223. Tan S, Hahn S, Benson S, et al. Metformin improves polycystic ovary syndrome symptoms irrespective of pre-treatment insulin resistance. Eur J Endocrinol. 2007;157:669–76.

224. Kolodziejczyk B, Duleba AJ, et al. Metformin therapy decreases hyperandrogenism and hyperinsulinemia in women with polycystic ovary syndrome. Fertil Steril. 2000;73:1149–54.

225. Martin KA, Chang RJ, Ehrmann DA, et al. Evaluation and treatment of hirsutism in premenopausal women: an endocrine society clinical practice guideline. J Clin Endocrinol Metab. 2008;93(4):1105–20.

226. Lizneva D, Gavrilova-Jordan L, Walker W, et al. Androgen excess: investigation and management. Best Pract Res Clin Obstet Gynaecol. 2016;37:98–118.

227. Liew SH. Laser hair removal: guidelines for management. Am J Clin Dermatol. 2002;3(2):107–15.

228. Wolf JE, Shander D, Huber F, et al. Randomized, double-blind clinical evaluation of the efficacy and safety of topical eflornithine HCl 13.9% cream in the treatment of women with facial hair. Int J Dermatol. 2007;46(1):94–8.

229. Blume-Peytavi U, Hahn S. Medical treatment of hirsutism. Dermatol Ther. 2008;21:329–39.

230. Malhotra B, Noveck R, Behr D, et al. Percutaneous absorption and pharmacokinetics of eflornithine HCL 13.9% cream in women with unwanted facial hair. J Clin Pharmacol. 2001;41:972–8.

231. Hickman JG, Huber F, Palmisano M. Human dermal safety studies with eflornitine HCL 13.9% cream (Vaniqa), a novel treatment for excessive facial hair. Curr Med Res Opin. 2001;16:235–44.

232. Prilepskaya VN, Serov VN, Zharov EV, et al. Effects of a phasic oral contraceptive containing desogestrel on facial seborrhea and acne. Contraception. 2003;68:239–45.

233. Grosman N, Hvidberg E, Schou J. The effect of estrogenic treatment on the acid mucopolysaccharide pattern in skin of mice. Acta Pharmacol Toxicol. 1971;30:458–64.

234. Uzuka M, Nakajima K, Ohta S, Mori Y. The mechanism of estrogen induced increase in hyaluronic acid biosynthesis, with special reference to estrogen receptor in the mouse skin. Biochim Biophys Acta. 1980;627:199–206.

235. Pierard-Franchimond C, Letane C, Goffin V, Pierard GE. Skin water-holding capacity and transdermal estrogen therapy for menopause: a pilot study. Maturitas. 1995;22:151–4.

236. Cakir GA, Erdogan FG, Gurler A. Isotretinoin treatment in nodulocystic acne with and without polycystic ovary syndrome: efficacy and determinants of relapse. Int J Dermatol. 2013;52:371–6.

237. Ibanez L, de Zegher F. Flutamide-metformin therapy to reduce fat mass in hyperinsulinemic ovarian hyperandrogenism: effects

in adolescents and in women on third generation oral contraception. J Clin Endocrinol Metab. 2003;88:4720–4.

238. Ibanez L, de Zegher F. Ethinylestradiol-drospirenone, flutamide-metformin, or both for adolescents and women with hyperinsulinemic hyperandrogenism: opposite effects on adipocytokines and body adiposity. J Clin Endocrinol Metab. 2004;89(4):1592–7.

239. Palep-Singh M, Mook K, Barth J, Balen A. An observational study of Yasmin in the management of women with polycystic ovary syndrome. J Fam Plann Reprod Health Care. 2004;30:163–5.

240. Lumachi F, Rondinone R. Use of cyproterone acetate, finasteride, and spironolactone to treat idiopathic hirsutism. Fertil Steril. 2003;79:942–6.

241. Cibula D, Hill M, Fanta M, et al. Does obesity diminish the positive effect of oral contraceptive treatment on hyperandrogenism in women with polycystic ovarian syndrome? Hum Reprod. 2001;16:940–4.

242. Holt VL, Cushing-Haugen KL, Daling JR. Body weight and risk of oral contraceptive failure. Obstet Gynecol. 2002;99:820–7.

243. Vexiau P, Chaspoux C, Boudou P, Fiet J, Jouanique C, Hardy N, et al. Effects of minoxidil 2% vs cyproterone acetate treatment on female androgenic alopecia: a controlled, 12 month randomized trial. Br J Dermatol. 2002;146:992–9.

244. Rogers NE, Avram MR. Medical treatments for male and female pattern hair loss. J Am Acad Dermatol. 2008;59:547–66.

245. Koulouri O, Conway GS. Management of hirsutism. BMJ. 2009;27:338.